MW01033967

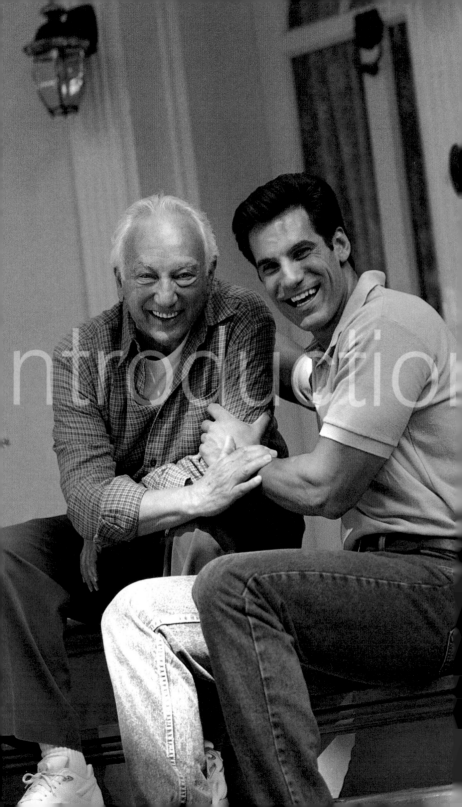

When you think about staying healthy, you probably think about making lifestyle changes to prevent conditions like cancer and heart disease. Keeping your bones healthy to prevent osteoporosis may not be at the top of your wellness list. But it should be. Here's why:

Osteoporosis is common. Osteoporosis is a condition in which the bones become weak and can break from a minor fall or, in serious cases, from a simple action such as a sneeze. Approximately 10 million Americans already have the disease. Another 34 million are at high risk for it. Being at risk for osteoporosis means you are more likely to get this disease. The U.S. Surgeon General reports that nearly half of all women older than 50 will break a bone because of osteoporosis. An estimated one in four men will too.

Osteoporosis is serious. Breaking a bone is serious, especially when you're older. Broken bones due to osteoporosis are most likely in the hip, spine and wrist, but any bone can be affected. It can cause severe pain that may not go away. For some people, it can cause a loss in height. Your posture may become stooped or hunched. This happens when the bones of the spine, called vertebrae, begin to break or collapse. Osteoporosis may even keep you from getting around easily and doing the things you enjoy. This can make you feel isolated and depressed. It can also lead to other health problems. Twenty percent of seniors who break a hip die within one year from problems related to the fracture itself or surgery to repair it. Many of those who survive need long-term nursing home care.

Osteoporosis is costly. In 2005, osteoporosis was responsible for an estimated two million fractures and $19 billion in costs. By 2025, experts predict that osteoporosis will be responsible for three million fractures and $25.3 billion in costs.

Osteoporosis can sneak up on you. You can't feel your bones growing weaker. You could have osteoporosis now or be at risk for it and not know it. Often, breaking a bone is the first clue that you have osteoporosis. Or maybe you notice that you are getting shorter or your upper spine is curving forward. At this point the disease is advanced. Fortunately, there are tests, called bone mineral density (BMD) tests, which can tell if you have osteoporosis before you have these symptoms. This makes it possible to treat the disease early to prevent fractures.

Boning Up on Osteoporosis will help you find out whether you are at risk for osteoporosis. It will also guide you in working with your healthcare providers to prevent or treat it. If you don't have osteoporosis, you can take steps now to prevent it. If you already have it, you should seek treatment. This can prevent further bone loss and decrease your chances of breaking a bone. It can also help you be more active and improve the quality of your life.

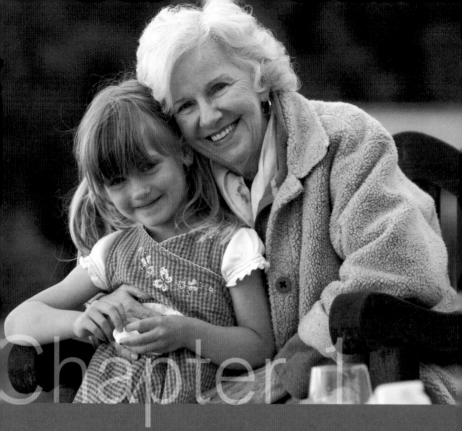

Chapter 1

Osteoporosis: What It Is and Who Is At Risk

Osteoporosis means "porous bone." If you looked at healthy bone under a microscope, you would see that parts of it look like a honeycomb. If you have osteoporosis, the holes and spaces in the honeycomb are much bigger than they are in healthy bone. This means your bones have lost density, or mass. It also means that the structure of your bone tissues has become abnormal. As your bones become less dense, they become weaker. For some people affected by the disease, simple activities such as lifting a child, bending down to pick up a newspaper or even sneezing can cause a bone to break.

Bone Basics

Because osteoporosis is a disease of the bones, it is important to know some basics about your bones.

Your bones are made up of three major components that make them both flexible and strong:

- Collagen, a protein that gives bones a flexible framework
- Calcium-phosphate mineral complexes that make bones hard and strong
- Living bone cells that remove and replace weakened sections of bone

How Bones Change and Grow

Throughout life, your skeleton loses old bone and forms new bone. Children and teenagers form new bone faster than they lose the old bone. In fact, even after they stop growing taller, young people continue to make more bone than they lose. This means their bones get denser and denser until they reach what experts call peak bone mass. This is the point when you have the greatest amount of bone you will ever have. It usually happens between the ages of 18 and 25.

After you reach peak bone mass, the balance between bone loss and bone formation might start to change. In other words, you may slowly start to lose more bone than you form. In midlife, bone loss usually speeds up in both men and women. For most women, bone loss increases after menopause, when estrogen levels drop sharply. In fact, in the five to seven years after menopause, women can lose up to 20 percent or more of their bone density.

Bone Tissue: Normal vs. osteoporotic bone

Normal bone 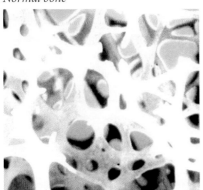   *Osteoporotic bone*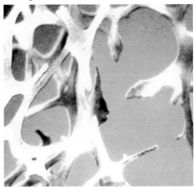

Risk Factors for Osteoporosis

- Being female
- Older age
- Family history of osteoporosis or broken bones
- Being small and thin
- Race/ethnicity such as Caucasian, Asian or Latino
- History of broken bones
- Menopause
- Low sex hormones
- Diet—especially one that is low in calcium and vitamin D
- Inactive lifestyle
- Smoking
- Alcohol abuse
- Certain medications such as steroid medications
- Certain diseases and conditions such as rheumatoid arthritis

These risk factors can help identify people who are more likely to get the disease. You can find out if you have osteoporosis by getting a bone mineral density (BMD) test (see pages 33-36). Ask your healthcare provider if you should have a BMD test.

Osteoporosis happens when you lose too much bone, make too little bone or both. The more bone you have at the time of peak bone mass, the better you will be protected against weak bones once bone loss begins.

Who Gets Osteoporosis: Factors That Put You at Risk

Osteoporosis can affect people of all ages, but it is far more common in older people than younger people. All of us lose some bone density as we age, but some of us lose more bone or lose it faster than others. It is not true that every older person gets osteoporosis, but it does become more common with age. About one-half of women in their 80s have it.

Osteoporosis is also more common in women than men. Eighty percent, or four out of five, of the 10 million Americans who have it are women. There are several reasons for this. Women have lighter, thinner bones to begin with. They also lose bone rapidly after menopause. In addition, women live longer than men, which gives them more years to develop the disease. In fact, a woman's risk of breaking a hip due to osteoporosis is equal to her combined risk of breast, ovarian and uterine cancer.

But this doesn't mean osteoporosis is just a woman's disease. When you think about it—if four out of five people with the disease are women—one out of five (two million people with osteoporosis) are men. A man older than 50 is more likely to break a bone due to osteoporosis than he is to get prostate cancer.

Age and Sex. Age and sex are just two factors that increase your risk of osteoporosis. While you have no control over some risk factors, there are others you can change. Many of the choices you make each day can affect your bones. By making healthier choices you can help to reduce your risk of osteoporosis as well as the painful fractures it can cause.

Family History. Research suggests that heredity and genetics play a major role in osteoporosis. If either of your parents had osteoporosis or a history of broken bones, you are more likely to get it too. Also, if one of your parents had a noticeable amount of height loss or a spine that curved forward, they may have had osteoporosis.

Low Body Weight/Being Small and Thin. Women and men with small bones are more likely than larger people to have osteoporosis. But that doesn't mean heavier or larger people can't get it.

Race and Ethnicity. While osteoporosis affects all races and ethnicities, people in the U.S. who are Caucasian or of Asian or Latino descent are more likely to develop osteoporosis than those of African heritage.

History of Broken Bones. People who have broken one or more bones during their adult years are at greater risk for osteoporosis.

Menopause. For most women, bone loss increases after menopause, when estrogen levels drop sharply (for more information, see page 30).

Low Sex Hormones
Estrogen Levels. In women, the sex hormone estrogen protects bones. If you are a woman and go through menopause early, your risk of osteoporosis increases. The same is true if you have your ovaries removed. That's because your ovaries produce most of your body's estrogen. In either of these cases, it's important to speak with your healthcare provider about steps to improve bone health. (See pages 42-45 to learn the latest about hormone replacement therapy.)

Missing Periods. If you are a young woman and don't have regular periods, this could mean low estrogen levels. There could be many reasons for this, such as exercising too much or eating so little that you become too thin. Other causes could include disorders of the ovaries or the pituitary, which is the gland in the brain that makes hormones. Regardless of the cause, loss of estrogen and extreme thinness can harm bone health. It can also affect other vital body systems. For these reasons, young women who don't have regular periods should speak to their healthcare provider.

Testosterone Levels. In men, testosterone protects bone. Estrogen levels in men are also important. Low levels of these hormones can lead to bone loss. A number of factors can cause levels to be low, including eating too little or drinking too much alcohol. A simple blood test can tell you if your hormone levels are normal.

Diet: How the Foods You Eat Can Affect Your Bones
Calcium. Calcium is a mineral that is important for healthy bones. It is a building block of bone. (For good sources of calcium, see pages 17-21.)

Vitamin D. Vitamin D is important because it helps your body use calcium. If you don't get enough vitamin D or if your body does not absorb it well, you are at much greater risk for bone loss and osteoporosis. (For more information on vitamin D, see page 20.)

Phosphorous. Like calcium, phosphorous is a part of the bones. Because this mineral is naturally present in many foods, most people get enough phosphorus. It is sometimes added to processed foods and soft drinks in the form of phosphate or phosphoric acid. While some experts say that Americans may be getting too much phosphorous, many experts believe that phosphorous intake is not a problem as long as people get enough calcium.

Other Minerals and Vitamins. Magnesium, vitamin K, vitamin B6 and vitamin B12 are some of the many minerals and vitamins that are important for bone

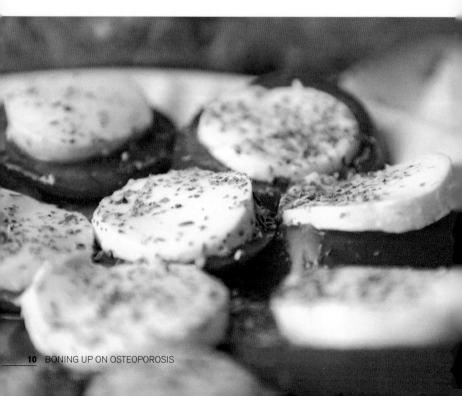

health. If you eat a well-balanced diet, you should be getting enough of these nutrients. Most experts recommend multivitamins or supplements for people who do not get what they need from foods.

Protein. Eating foods that supply protein is important for your health. But a very high protein diet, particularly animal protein, causes a loss of calcium through the kidneys. You can make up for this calcium loss by getting enough calcium to meet your body's needs.

Caffeine. Found naturally in coffee and tea, caffeine is often added to soft drinks. Caffeine appears to decrease calcium absorption. One study suggests that drinking 330 mg of caffeine, or about four cups of coffee, daily increases the risk of fractures. You can also make up for calcium loss due to caffeine by getting enough calcium to meet your body's needs.

Soft Drinks. Some people are concerned that the phosphorous and/or caffeine in certain soft drinks may harm bone health. Other experts suggest the harm to bone is caused by people substituting soft drinks for milk and calcium-fortified juices.

Sodium (salt). Eating foods that have a lot of sodium may decrease your body's ability to retain calcium. Eating too much sodium is bad for your bones and can cause bone loss. Try cooking without adding extra salt, and limit the salty snacks and processed foods that you eat.

Medications That Can Cause Bone Loss*

Aluminum-containing antacids

Antiseizure medications (only some) such as Dilantin® or Phenobarbital

Aromatase inhibitors such as Arimidex®, Aromasin® and Femara®

Cancer chemotherapeutic drugs

Cyclosporine A and FK506 (Tacrolimus)

Glucocorticoids such as cortisone and prednisone

Gonadotropin releasing hormone (GnRH) such as Lupron® and Zoladex®

Heparin

Lithium

Medroxyprogesterone acetate for contraception (Depo-Provera®)

Methotrexate

Proton pump inhibitors (PPIs) such as Nexium®, Prevacid® and Prilosec®

Selective serotonin reuptake inhibitors (SSRIs) such as Lexapro®, Prozac® and Zoloft®

Tamoxifen® (premenopausal use)

Thiazolidenediones such as Actos® and Avandia®

Thyroid hormones in excess

This list may not include all medications that cause bone loss.

Osteoporosis and Steroid Medications

Glucocorticoids (also known as corticosteroids or steroids) are powerful medications that relieve inflammation. They are often referred to as steroids and should not be confused with anabolic steroids. Anabolic steroids are male sex hormones that some athletes use illegally to build muscle.

Steroids are much like certain hormones made by your own body. Healthcare providers prescribe them for many conditions, including arthritis, asthma, Crohn's disease, allergies and lupus. These medications are also used along with other medications to treat cancer and support organ transplants. Common steroid medications are cortisone, prednisone and methylprednisolone.

People of all ages can lose bone and develop fractures if they take large doses of steroids. People whose adrenal glands make too much of the hormone cortisol (a condition called Cushing's syndrome) may also develop osteoporosis.

While steroid medicines increase your risk of osteoporosis, they can be life-saving treatments for some conditions. If you take steroid medications for more than a few weeks, you should take steps to prevent bone loss. Taking steroids in a dose of 5 mg or more per day for more than three months increases your risk of bone loss and can lead to osteoporosis.

Talk with your healthcare provider about prescribing the smallest dose of medicine for the shortest period of time to control your symptoms. While taking steroids, it is especially important to get enough calcium and vitamin D. It is also important to exercise and not smoke. You may also want to ask your healthcare provider if you need a bone mineral density (BMD) test.

Spinach. Spinach contains high levels of oxalate. Oxalate prevents the body from absorbing calcium from spinach. The body can absorb calcium found in most other green vegetables such as broccoli and kale.

Wheat Bran. 100% wheat bran is the only food that appears to reduce the absorption of calcium in other foods that are eaten at the same time. If you are taking calcium supplements, you may want to take your supplement two or more hours before or after eating any foods with 100% wheat bran. (For good sources of calcium, see pages 17-21.)

Other Factors That Affect Bone Health
Inactive Lifestyle. People who are bedridden, are inactive or do not exercise are at high risk of osteoporosis. Certain kinds of regular exercise can help keep your bones strong. (To learn more about exercise, see page 23-26 and Chapter 6.)

Smoking. Smoking is bad for your bones in many ways. The chemicals in cigarettes are bad for your bone cells. Smoking also might make it harder to absorb calcium. For women, smoking can prevent estrogen from protecting the bones.

Alcohol Abuse. Drinking heavily can reduce bone formation. In many cases, people who drink too much do not get enough calcium. Drinking may also affect your body's calcium supply. In addition, drinking too much is bad for your overall health and can make you more likely to fall. This is how many people break bones. Alcohol in smaller amounts, however, does not harm bone health. This usually means no more than three drinks a day.

Medications. Some medications can be harmful to your bones, especially if you take them at high doses or for a long time. One of the riskiest types of medications for bones is steroid medications. Many people take these medications to ease inflammation in conditions like rheumatoid arthritis or asthma. It's important to talk with your healthcare provider about the risks and benefits of any medications you take and about how they may affect your bones. Do not stop any treatment or change the dose of your medications unless your healthcare provider says it's safe to do so. (For a list of medications that can cause bone loss, see page 11; for more information about steroid medications, see page 12.)

Diseases and Conditions That Cause Bone Loss

There are many health problems that can harm your bones and increase your risk of osteoporosis. These include:

Anorexia Nervosa and Other Eating Disorders. Anorexia nervosa is a major risk factor for osteoporosis. In women with anorexia nervosa,

Are Osteoporosis and Osteoarthritis Connected?

Many people confuse osteoporosis and osteoarthritis. That's probably because the word osteoporosis is very similar to osteoarthritis (OA). Osteoarthritis is the most common form of arthritis. Osteoarthritis is a disease of thinning joint cartilage. Aside from their names, osteoporosis and osteoarthritis have little in common. Although people can have both of these diseases, osteoporosis and osteoarthritis have very different causes and treatments.

But osteoarthritis is just one of many diseases that affect the joints and surrounding tissues. These types of diseases are known as arthritis. And some forms of arthritis are associated with an increased risk for osteoporosis. One example is the second most common form of arthritis, rheumatoid arthritis (RA). Steroid medications used to treat it, as well as the condition on its own, can increase the risk of osteoporosis.

Medical Conditions That Can Lead to Osteoporosis*

AIDS/HIV

Ankylosing spondylitis

Blood and bone marrow disorders

Breast cancer

Cushing's syndrome

Eating disorders

Emphysema

Female athlete triad

Gastrectomy

Gastrointestinal bypass procedures

Hyperparathyroidism

Hyperthyroidism

Idiopathic scoliosis

Inflammatory bowel disease

Diabetes mellitus

Kidney disease

Lupus

Lymphoma and leukemia

Malabsorption syndromes (examples are celiac disease and Crohn's disease)

Multiple myeloma

Multiple sclerosis

Organ transplants

Parkinson's disease

Poor diet

Post-polio syndrome

Premature menopause

Prostate cancer

Rheumatoid arthritis

Severe liver disease (including biliary cirrhosis)

Spinal cord injuries

Stroke (CVA)

Thalassemia

Thyrotoxicosis

Weight loss

This list may not include all conditions that cause bone loss.

estrogen levels decrease to such an extent that menstrual periods either become irregular or stop. This drop in estrogen causes bone loss. A number of other complex changes occur in the body, and these are also harmful to the bones. Although more common in teenage girls and young women, men can also have eating disorders, and they too are at great risk for bone loss and osteoporosis.

Depression. Research suggests a link between depression and low bone density or osteoporosis. More studies will help us to better understand the relationship between these two conditions.

Hyperparathyroidism. This is a condition in which the parathyroid glands (two pairs of small glands located near the thyroid in the neck) produce too much parathyroid hormone (PTH). Having too much PTH causes bone loss. This condition is more common in women after menopause. A simple blood test can tell your healthcare provider if this is a problem.

Hyperthyroidism. In people with this condition, the thyroid gland produces too much thyroid hormone. This can lead to weak muscles and fragile bones. The same thing can happen if you have an underactive thyroid and take too much thyroid hormone medication.

Multiple Myeloma. This is a cancer of the bone marrow. Its first symptoms may be back pain and fractures of the vertebrae. Blood and urine tests can detect the problem. Other forms of cancer that affect bones or bone marrow can also cause fractures.

Rheumatoid Arthritis (RA). People with rheumatoid arthritis are at increased risk for osteoporosis. In addition, RA is often treated with steroids which further increases the risk.

Inflammatory Bowel Disease (IBD). There are different types of IBD including Crohn's disease and ulcerative colitis. Steroid medications are commonly used to treat these conditions. People with IBD may also have trouble absorbing calcium and vitamin D.

Celiac Disease. People with celiac disease have trouble digesting foods with gluten. Gluten is found in grains such as wheat, rye and barley. People with this condition also have problems absorbing nutrients, including calcium and vitamin D.

Organ Transplants. People who have organ transplants must take medications to prevent their bodies from rejecting their new organs. Some of these drugs can weaken bones.

Weight Loss. Losing weight can cause bone loss. Many serious conditions such as heart disease and diabetes are associated with obesity and excess weight. Fortunately, you can protect your bones while losing weight by exercising regularly and eating a healthy diet that provides enough calcium and vitamin D.

Loss of Height. Vertebral (spine) fractures cause height loss and kyphosis. Kyphosis is an abnormal forward curvature of the spine. When there is no pain, these fractures often go unnoticed until a person becomes aware that a significant loss of height of an inch or more has occurred.

Other Diseases and Conditions. Many other health problems can also affect the bones. Some of these include genetic disorders and diseases of the kidneys, lungs or digestive system. With proper treatment, most people can live well with these diseases. Living well also involves taking good care of your bones.

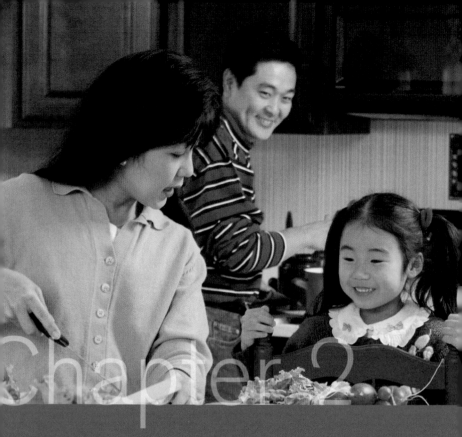

Preventing Bone Loss at Any Age

You're never too young or too old to improve the health of your bones. Osteoporosis prevention should begin in childhood. But it shouldn't stop there. Whatever your age, the habits you adopt now can affect your bone health for the rest of your life.

The Recipe for Healthy Bones

No matter what your age, the recipe for bone health is simple for both men and women:

- Get enough calcium and vitamin D
- Exercise regularly
- Make healthy lifestyle choices
- Talk to your healthcare provider about your bone health

In this chapter we'll discuss each of these four ingredients. Then we'll offer some guidance for building—or keeping—healthy bones at your specific stage of life.

Eat Healthy Foods

Most foods contain vitamins, minerals and other nutrients that help keep your body healthy. Your body needs these nutrients to work properly. Eating plenty of fruits and vegetables benefits your body in many ways, including your bones. Two nutrients that are of special importance to your bones are calcium and vitamin D.

Calcium

Calcium is an essential nutrient because it provides the material for building new bone. It's important throughout your life, particularly when you are growing. For women, it is especially important if you are pregnant or breastfeeding. Dairy products (low-fat or non-fat milk, yogurt and cheese) are good sources of calcium. So are products that have calcium added, such as certain cereals, soy milk and juices. You can get calcium in smaller amounts from broccoli, certain leafy green vegetables and soybeans. If you drink soy milk that is fortified with calcium, be sure to shake the container thoroughly as calcium can settle to the bottom.

If you are lactose intolerant (which means that you have trouble digesting milk due to a shortage of a protein called lactase), you might be able to eat lactose-free dairy products or those with added lactase. Another option is to eat other calcium-rich foods and ones that have added calcium.

If you don't get enough calcium from food (check calcium calculator, page 20, to find out) consider taking a calcium supplement. The amount of supplement you need depends on how much calcium you get each day from the foods you eat. It's important not to get too much calcium, because that can be harmful, too.

Calcium exists in nature only in combination with other substances called

DOs and DON'Ts for Choosing a Calcium Supplement

The following DOs and DON'Ts can help you in choosing and using a calcium supplement. If you still have concerns about the right supplement or amount, speak with your healthcare provider.

Do

DO ask your pharmacist to recommend a calcium supplement. Pay close attention to the serving size and amount of calcium per serving.

DO read the package label. It will tell you the amount of elemental calcium—how much calcium the supplement provides—and how many doses or pills you must take to get that amount.

DO ask your pharmacist about possible interactions between calcium supplements and any medications you take.

DO take supplements with food whenever possible. Except for calcium citrate, calcium supplements are better absorbed by your body when taken with food. You can take your supplement during or right after a meal or snack.

DO consider foods that have calcium added instead of supplements. Some brands of cereal and fruit juice have calcium added.

DO check with your healthcare provider or pharmacist if you take 40 mg or more of proton pump inhibitors (PPIs) daily. Examples of PPIs include Nexium®, Prevacid® and Prilosec®. Because these medications block stomach acid, your body may better absorb calcium citrate supplements. Calcium citrate, unlike other calcium supplements, doesn't need stomach acid for absorption.

Don't

DON'T buy a supplement from unrefined oyster shell, bone meal or dolomite unless the label states "purified" or has the USP (United States Pharmacopeia) symbol. These may contain lead and other toxic metals.

DON'T take all of your calcium at once. If possible, spread it out over two or three doses per day. Your body absorbs calcium best in amounts of 600 mg or less.

DON'T take more calcium than you need. Estimate the amount of calcium you get from your diet. Extra calcium from supplements won't help, and it might cause problems such as kidney stones in certain individuals.

DON'T take an iron supplement at the same time as your calcium supplement. Calcium may prevent your body from properly using the iron.

DON'T use antacids containing aluminum as a calcium supplement. Large doses of aluminum can harm bone. Using an antacid with calcium carbonate, as long as it doesn't contain aluminum, is fine.

compounds. Several different calcium compounds are used in supplements, including calcium carbonate, calcium citrate, calcium lactate and calcium phosphate. These compounds contain different amounts of elemental calcium, which is the actual amount of calcium in the supplement. It is important to read the product label carefully to determine how much elemental calcium is in the supplement and how many doses or pills to take. When reading the label, pay close attention to the "amount per serving" and "serving size."

Calcium supplements are available without a prescription in a wide range of preparations (including chewable and liquid) and in various strengths. Many people ask which calcium supplement they should take. The best supplement is the one that meets an individual's needs based on tolerance, convenience, cost and availability.

Calcium and Vitamin D* Recommendations

Children and Adolescents	Calcium (Daily)	Vitamin D (Daily)
1 through 3 years	500 mg	200 IU**
4 through 8 years	800 mg	200 IU**
9 through 18 years	1,300 mg	200 IU**
Adult Women and Men	Calcium (Daily)	Vitamin D_3 (Daily)*
19 through 49 years	1,000 mg	400-800 IU
50 years and over	1,200 mg	800-1,000 IU
Pregnant and Breastfeeding Women	Calcium (Daily)	Vitamin D_3 (Daily)*
18 years and under	1,300 mg	400-800 IU
19 years and over	1,000 mg	400-800 IU

Vitamin D_3 is also called cholecalciferol; vitamin D_2 is also called ergocalciferol.

*When available, a supplement of vitamin D_3 is preferred over vitamin D_2 to protect bone health.

**The National Osteoporosis Foundation does not have specific vitamin D recommendations for these age groups. These are the recommendations of the Institute of Medicine of the National Academies and National Institutes of Health, Office of Dietary Supplements.

Calculate Your Calcium. Are you getting enough calcium in your diet? Your calcium needs vary at different times in your life. Here's a general guide.

Try keeping a diary of all the foods you eat for a week or two. Then use the results of a typical day to fill out this calcium calculator and compare your results to "Calcium and Vitamin D Recommendations" (see page 19). If you find that you fall short, select a calcium supplement to make up the difference.

Product	Servings/day		Estimated calcium/ serving, in mg		Calcium, in mg
Milk (8 oz.)	_____	x	300	=	_____
Yogurt (8 oz.)	_____	x	400	=	_____
Cheese (1 oz.)	_____	x	200	=	_____
Fortified foods or juices	_____	x	80 to 1000*	=	_____
Estimated total from other foods with smaller amounts of calcium					_____ 250
Total daily calcium intake				=	_____

Calcium content of fortified food varies. Check package label.

How Much Vitamin D Do I Need?

NOF recommends getting between 800 and 1,000 international units (IU) of vitamin D_3 daily for most people age 50 and older. Some people may need more. Adults under 50 should get between 400 and 800 IU of vitamin D_3 daily. Supplements of vitamin D are available as either vitamin D_2 or D_3. Vitamin D_3 is the better choice to protect your bones. It is also called cholecalciferol.

Vitamin D

Your body needs vitamin D to absorb calcium. Your skin makes vitamin D when it is exposed to the sun. In fact, sunlight is the main source of vitamin D for many people, but we know that getting sun is a risk factor for skin cancers and other skin diseases. In some people, vitamin D levels can remain low despite sun exposure. People who live in northern latitudes are not able to produce vitamin D from the sun during the winter months.

Vitamin D is usually added to the milk you buy at the grocery store (but not to other milk-based products, like cheese, yogurt and butter). Liver, fatty fish and egg yolks also contain vitamin D. It is very difficult to get enough of this nutrient from food, so many people will need to take a multivitamin or a vitamin D supplement. Many calcium supplements also contain vitamin D, but it is

Calcium Content of Foods

Food item	Serving size	Estimated calcium content in milligrams (mg)
Milk		
Whole, low-fat or skim	8 oz. (1 cup)	300
Yogurt and ice-cream		
Plain yogurt, fat-free or low-fat	8 oz. (1 cup)	415
Fruit yogurt, low-fat	8 oz. (1 cup)	345
Frozen yogurt, vanilla, soft-serve	8 oz. (1 cup)	205
Ice-cream, low-fat or high-fat	8 oz. (1 cup)	140-210
Cheese		
American	1 oz.	175
Cheddar, shredded	1 oz.	205
Cottage cheese, 1% milk fat	1 cup	140
Mozzarella, part skim	1 oz.	205
Parmesan, grated	1 tbsp.	70
Ricotta, part skim	4 oz. (1/2 cup)	335
Swiss	1 oz.	220-270
Fish and shellfish (canned)		
Sardines, canned in oil with bones	3 oz.	325
Salmon, pink, canned with bones	3 oz.	180
Shrimp, canned	3 oz.	125
Vegetables		
Bok choy (Chinese cabbage), raw	8 oz. (1 cup)	75
Broccoli, cooked & drained	8 oz. (1 cup)	60
Kale, cooked	8 oz. (1 cup)	95
Soybeans, mature, cooked & drained	8 oz. (1 cup)	175
Turnip greens, fresh, cooked & drained	8 oz. (1 cup)	200
Fruits		
Oranges	1 whole	50
Dried figs	2 figs	55
Fortified foods		
Fruit juice with added calcium	6 oz.	200-345
Cereal with added calcium (without milk)	1 cup	100-1,000
Tofu prepared with calcium	4 oz. (1/2 cup)	205
Soy milk with added calcium	8 oz. (1 cup)	80-500

The calcium content listed for most foods is estimated and can vary due to multiple factors such as fortification and fat content.

When a serving of milk says it contains 30% calcium, how do I know how much calcium is in that serving?

The percent Daily Values (DV) on the food label can help you determine whether a food is high or low in a nutrient. In general, 5% DV or less is low in a nutrient, while 20% DV or more is high. Daily Values are available on the "Nutrition Facts" panel on food labels, which should be read carefully because the percent DV is based on one serving of food.

The DV for calcium is based on 1,000 mg daily. Therefore, a serving of milk with a DV of 30% calcium means that it contains 300 mg of calcium. A serving of food with a DV of 20% calcium means it contains 200 mg of calcium and 10% means it contains 100 mg of calcium.

In the case of vitamin D, the DV is based on 400 IU daily. Therefore a serving of food with 50% vitamin D has 200 IU of vitamin D. A serving of food with 25% vitamin D has 100 IU of vitamin D. There are few food sources for vitamin D, so unless an item has been fortified with vitamin D, most food labels do not list the percent of the DV of vitamin D.

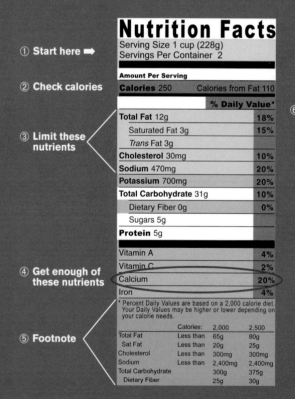

① Start here ➡

② Check calories

③ Limit these nutrients

④ Get enough of these nutrients

⑤ Footnote

⑥ Quick guide to % DV

5% or less is low

20% or more is high

Nutrition Facts

Serving Size 1 cup (228g)
Servings Per Container 2

Amount Per Serving

Calories 250   Calories from Fat 110

	% Daily Value*
Total Fat 12g	18%
Saturated Fat 3g	15%
Trans Fat 3g	
Cholesterol 30mg	10%
Sodium 470mg	20%
Potassium 700mg	20%
Total Carbohydrate 31g	10%
Dietary Fiber 0g	0%
Sugars 5g	
Protein 5g	
Vitamin A	4%
Vitamin C	2%
Calcium	20%
Iron	4%

* Percent Daily Values are based on a 2,000 calorie diet. Your Daily Values may be higher or lower depending on your calorie needs.

	Calories:	2,000	2,500
Total Fat	Less than	65g	80g
Sat Fat	Less than	20g	25g
Cholesterol	Less than	300mg	300mg
Sodium	Less than	2,400mg	2,400mg
Total Carbohydrate		300g	375g
Dietary Fiber		25g	30g

not necessary to take vitamin D and calcium supplements together.

Your healthcare provider can run a simple blood test that can tell if you're getting enough vitamin D for healthy bones. If you aren't, your healthcare provider may prescribe extra doses of vitamin D until your blood levels increase. Your healthcare provider may need to repeat the test a few times until your blood levels of vitamin D are normal.

Exercise Regularly

You know that your muscles get bigger and stronger when you use them. Bones are similar; they get stronger and denser when you make them work. And "work" for bones means handling impact, the weight of your body, or more resistance. Currently, we know the most about two types of exercises that are important for building and maintaining bone density. These are:

Weight-bearing, impact exercises. These exercises include activities that make you move against gravity while being upright, such as fast walking, running, stair climbing and playing soccer. Biking and swimming are not weight-bearing exercises so they don't help your bones as much. If you like these activities, try to add in other activities that work your bones.

Resistance/strengthening exercises. Resistance or strengthening exercise is when you move your body, a weight, or some other resistance against gravity. This can include functional movements, such as standing and rising up on your toes, or resistance/strengthening exercises such as lifting weights, using elastic exercise bands, weight machines or lifting your own body weight.

Your program may also include the following types of exercises:

Balance exercises. Exercises that strengthen your legs and challenge your balance, such as Tai Chi, can decrease your risk of falls.

Posture exercises. Exercises that improve your posture and reduce rounded or "sloping" shoulders can help you decrease the risk of fractures, especially in the spine.

Functional exercises. Exercises that improve how well you move can help you in everyday activities and decrease your risk of falls and fractures. For example, if you have trouble getting up from a chair or climbing stairs, you should do functional exercises.

Refer to Chapter 6 for specific exercises that can help you strengthen your hips and spine, improve your balance and posture and how you move in your everyday life.

If you can't do high-impact weight-bearing activities, try lower-impact ones. For example, try walking or stair-climbing instead of jogging. If you haven't exercised regularly for a while, check with your healthcare provider before beginning a new exercise program—particularly if you have health problems such as heart disease, diabetes or high blood pressure. Once you have your healthcare provider's approval, start slowly.

If you have already had spine fractures from osteoporosis, be very careful to avoid activities that require reaching down, bending forward, rapid twisting motions, heavy lifting and those that increase your chance of a fall.

How Much Exercise Should I Do?

Weight-bearing, impact exercises should be done for 30 total minutes on most days of the week. You can do 30 minutes at one time or break it up during the day. For example, 3 sessions for 10 minutes each will provide the same bone benefit as one 30-minute session. If you can't fit 10 minutes in, spread your impact exercises through your day by taking the stairs or by parking farther from the store or work.

Resistance/strengthening exercises should be done two to three days per week. You should aim for one exercise for each major muscle group for a total of 8-12 exercises. You should do one or two sets of 8 to 10 repetitions for each exercise. If you lift a weight 10 times in a row and then stop, you have completed one set of 10 repetitions. If you can't do 8 in a row, the weight is too heavy or resistance is too much. If you can do more than 10 in a row, you should probably increase the weight or resistance. If you have osteoporosis or are frail, you may be able to do 10 to 15 repetitions of a lighter weight. If you're at high risk of having a fracture, you should work with a physical therapist to develop a safe strength training program.

If you don't have much time for strengthening/resistance training, do small amounts at a time. You can do just one body part each day. For example do arms one day, legs the next and trunk the next. You can also spread these exercises out during your normal day.

Balance, posture and functional exercises can be done every day. You may focus on one area more than the others. If you have fallen or lose your balance, spend time doing the balance exercises. If you are getting rounded shoulders, work more on the posture exercises. If you have trouble climbing stairs or getting up from the couch, do more functional exercises. You can also perform these exercises at one time or spread them throughout your day.

As you get started, your muscles may feel sore for a day or two after you exercise. If soreness lasts longer, you may be working too hard and need to ease up. Exercises should be done in a pain-free range of motion.

Healthy Bones Exercise Schedule

Your healthy bones exercise week may look like one of the following two examples. Adjust your schedule to fit your specific needs and your lifestyle.

Exercise	Sun	Mon	Tues	Wed	Thurs	Fri	Sat
Weight-bearing, impact exercise	30 min.	30 min.		30 min.		30 min.	30 min.
Resistance/ strengthening exercise			8-12 types		8-12 types		
Balance, posture, and functional (Chap. 6)	✓	✓	✓	✓	✓	✓	✓

Exercise	Sun	Mon	Tues	Wed	Thurs	Fri	Sat
Weight-bearing, impact exercise	30 min.		30 min.	30 min.	30 min.		30 min.
Resistance/ strengthening exercise	4 arm*	4 leg	3 trunk	4 arm*	4 leg	3 trunk	
Balance, posture, and functional (Chap. 6)	✓	✓	✓	✓	✓	✓	✓

Even though arm exercises are not included in this booklet, they are part of a complete resistance/strengthening program.

If you've had a fracture or have osteoporosis or low bone density, work with a physical therapist to choose the best exercise and learn the correct exercise form.

All individuals should check with their healthcare provider before beginning an exercise program. If you have any chest pain, stop exercising and see your healthcare provider before exercising again.

Which Exercise Is Best?

The activities in Group 1 are the most effective for building bone. If you already have low bone mass, osteoporosis or are frail, choose safer options from Groups 2, 3 and 4.

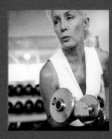

GROUP 1: WEIGHT-BEARING HIGH-IMPACT/RESISTANCE ACTIVITIES

- Aerobic Dancing
- Basketball
- Dancing
- Field Hockey
- Gymnastics
- Hiking
- Jogging or Running
- Jumping Rope
- Lacrosse
- Racquet Sports
- Soccer
- Stair Climbing
- Tennis
- Volleyball
- Weight Lifting or Resistance Training

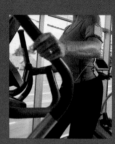

GROUP 2: WEIGHT-BEARING LOW-IMPACT ACTIVITIES:

- Cross-Country Ski Machines (avoid if you have balance problems and are at risk of falls)
- Downhill and Cross-Country Skiing (avoid if you have balance problems and are at risk of falls)
- Elliptical Training Machines
- Low Impact Aerobics
- Stair-Step Machines
- Treadmill Walking
- Walking

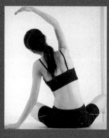

GROUP 3: NON-IMPACT/BALANCE/POSTURE/FUNCTIONAL EXERCISES

- Balance Training Exercises
- Functional Exercises
- Pilates (avoid forward-bending exercises)
- Posture Exercises
- Tai Chi
- Yoga (avoid forward-bending exercises)

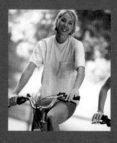

GROUP 4: NON-WEIGHT-BEARING NON-IMPACT ACTIVITIES

- Bicycling and Indoor Cycling
- Deep-Water Walking
- Stretching and Flexibility Exercises (avoid forward-bending exercises)
- Swimming
- Water Aerobics

Healthy Lifestyle Choices

Lifestyle habits like smoking and drinking alcohol can affect your bones. If you drink, do so in moderation. Heavy drinking reduces bone formation. It might also affect your body's calcium supply. Drinking alcohol can also make you more likely to fall, which is how many people break bones. Moderate drinking, however, does not harm bones. But if you drink more than two alcoholic drinks a day you need to be concerned.

If you smoke, stop. If you don't smoke, don't start. Smoking is bad for your bones for many reasons. The nicotine and other chemicals in cigarettes are toxic to bone cells. Smoking might also make it harder for you to absorb calcium. In addition, smoking decreases the ability of estrogen to help protect bones in women. Finally, smoking can make exercise harder because it stresses the heart and lungs. It's no surprise, then, that researchers say smokers are more likely than nonsmokers to break bones.

Talk With Your Healthcare Provider

If your healthcare provider hasn't talked to you about your bone health, it is time for you to bring it up. The two of you can develop a plan for protecting your bones.

Depending on your age and other risk factors, your healthcare provider may recommend a bone mineral density (BMD) test. (We'll discuss that further in Chapter 3.) The test will tell if you have osteoporosis or are at risk for developing it. If the test shows you are losing bone density, your healthcare provider may prescribe medication to prevent or treat osteoporosis. These drugs fall into two main categories: antiresorptives and anabolics. Antiresorptives slow bone loss.

Questions to Ask Your Healthcare Provider

Your healthcare provider can answer your questions about bone health. Here are some questions you might want to ask:

- How can I prevent osteoporosis?
- How can I protect my bones?
- Which are the best exercises for me?
- How much calcium and vitamin D do I need?
- Should I take a supplement? If so, which type is best for me and how much should I take?
- Can any of the medications I take harm my bones? If so, what can I do?
- Do I need a bone mineral density (BMD) test?
- Should I take a medication to prevent osteoporosis? If so, what are my options? What are the benefits and risks of these medications?

Anabolics build bones. You can learn more about them in Chapter 4 on treatment.

What You Can Do Now at Each Stage of Life

While the same basic recipe for bone health will serve you well throughout life, there are some specific things you can and should do at each stage of life. Find the stage where you are and get started now.

Childhood Through Adulthood: Building Strong Bones

Building strong bones when you are young can help you avoid osteoporosis later in life. Children and teenagers form new bone faster than they lose old bone. Their bones get denser and denser until they reach what experts call peak bone mass. This is the point when you have the greatest amount of bone you will ever have. It usually occurs between the ages of 18 and 25.

To help build strong bones, it is important to be physically active throughout childhood, the teen years and young adulthood. Children and teens should get at least one hour of physical activity every day. Adults should get at least 30 minutes of moderate physical activity daily. Activities such as jumping rope, running and playing sports are fun and make bones stronger. Lifting weights, using weight machines or taking certain exercise classes builds both muscles and bones.

Eating properly and getting enough calcium are also important at these stages of your life. Avoid drinking sodas in place of milk or calcium-fortified juices. If you are a teen or young adult, avoid excessive dieting. Becoming too thin now could affect your bones for the rest of your life. Smoking and drinking too much alcohol can also harm your bones now and in the future.

When Kids Get Osteoporosis

There is no generally accepted definition of osteoporosis in children. Low bone density in children is most commonly due to other medical conditions or medications used to treat certain diseases. Sometimes there is no known cause for low bone density in children. In some cases, children who have many fractures have an underlying problem with their bones called osteogenesis imperfecta. This disease is different from osteoporosis and can be diagnosed with a blood test.

A rare form of osteoporosis, called idiopathic juvenile osteoporosis, affects children between the ages of 1 and 13. Its cause is unknown. Children with this condition tend to have fractures, particularly of the legs and spine. Treatment includes calcium and vitamin D and, in some cases, medication. Fortunately, this type of osteoporosis usually goes away at adolescence. Experts are not certain whether this condition will affect bone health later in life.

Steroid medications can also put children at risk of losing bone density. Steroids are strong medicines used to treat diseases such as arthritis, asthma and Crohn's disease. (See Osteoporosis and Steroid Medications on page 12.) If your child must take one of these drugs, speak with his or her healthcare provider about bone protection. The Food and Drug Administration (FDA) has not approved the use of osteoporosis medications in children.

Young Adulthood to Middle Age: Maintaining Peak Bone Mass
Once you are 25, your bones are probably as strong as they will ever be. If you have a healthy lifestyle and if you are a woman with regular periods, you probably won't lose much bone over the next 20 years. But if you are inactive or don't get enough calcium and vitamin D, you can start losing bone. Bone loss can also happen if sex hormone levels are low or if you have a disease that causes bone loss. (See Medical Conditions That Can Lead to Osteoporosis, page 14.) In these cases, it is especially important to start a program to prevent bone loss.

Teenagers who use Depo-Provera® for birth control may be at risk for bone loss and osteoporosis later in life. The Food and Drug Administration (FDA) advises women that Depo-Provera® should not be used longer than two years if there are other birth control choices.

Some experts are concerned that even oral contraceptives (birth control pills) may have negative effects on bone, such as limiting bone size. For teenagers, this may affect bone strength later in life. Talk to your healthcare provider about the possible benefits and risks of taking oral contraceptives.

If you are pregnant or breastfeeding, it is especially important to get the calcium and vitamin D you need. The need is greatest for teenagers who become pregnant, because they must provide for their own growing bones and those of their baby. So, for teenage pregnancies, the effects on future bone health are not certain. Women who have one or more pregnancies and/or miscarriages as an adult experience no lasting harm to their bones.

Healthy lifestyle choices continue to be important during this stage of your life. Drinking too much alcohol or smoking can lead to bone loss. Exercise and a proper diet can help keep bones strong. If you have young children or grandchildren, now is the time to help them develop healthy habits to protect their bones too.

Middle Age and Beyond: Preventing Bone Loss Later in Life
In your 30s and 40s you may begin to lose bone, especially if you have certain illnesses, take medicines that cause bone loss or have other risk factors. (For information on risk factors, see Chapter 1.) Women have more wrist fractures in their 40s than men. This may be a sign of bone loss even before menopause.

WHAT WOMEN NEED TO KNOW
Menopause: A Time for Action
At some point, all women go through menopause. At first monthly periods become less regular. This is called perimenopause. A woman reaches menopause when her periods stop completely. This transition happens naturally over time. In some women it takes less than a year. In others it can take two or more years. During this time, you may feel many physical and emotional changes. Or you may feel no symptoms at all.

Menopause happens when the ovaries stop producing estrogen. If you have your ovaries removed, menopause happens abruptly. Either way it happens, the result is the same: low estrogen levels, which can lead to bone loss. In some women, bone loss is rapid and severe.

The amount of bone you have at menopause and how fast you lose it afterwards are the two most important factors in determining if you will develop osteoporosis. When you reach menopause, you may want to ask your healthcare provider about whether you should have a BMD test at this time (see pages 33-36). With BMD tests, it is possible to tell if you are at risk for osteoporosis. Knowing this can help you begin treatment before you lose too much bone.

In women, bone loss is most rapid during the first few years after menopause. But it continues throughout life. Bone loss at the hip can speed up in your 70s or 80s. This may be due to less physical activity and other changes in the way your body breaks down and builds bone. Most men do not begin to lose bone until their 50s, and their rate of bone loss is slower than women's. However, men can lose a lot of bone later in life and are also at risk for fractures.

It's important for older women and men to get enough calcium (1,200 mg/day) and vitamin D (800-1,000 IU/day). Staying active is essential for keeping toned muscles, flexible joints, strong bones and good balance.

If you already have osteoporosis, you should work with your healthcare provider to find the best way to treat it and prevent further bone loss. (For more on treatment, see Chapter 4.) You should also take steps to reduce your risk of falls, which can lead to broken bones.

If you have risk factors, or aren't sure, it's important to speak with your healthcare provider about the best ways to protect your bones. BMD tests can tell if you have low bone density and if you need medical treatment.

WHAT MEN NEED TO KNOW
Men Get Osteoporosis Too

If you think you can't get osteoporosis because you are a man, think again. Although women are at greater risk, osteoporosis can affect men, too. As the population ages, more and more men will get the disease. Here are some facts and statistics:

- In American men over age 50, two million already have osteoporosis. Another 12 million are at risk.
- One in every four men over age 50 is at risk for an osteoporosis-related fracture.
- Each year, approximately 80,000 men will fracture a hip.
- Men are also more likely than women to die within a year from problems related to a hip fracture.
- Men can develop painful spinal fractures but usually at a later age than women.

Factors such as using steroid medications, not exercising, smoking, drinking too much alcohol or having low testosterone levels put you at risk. So does having other medical problems such as chronic kidney, lung or gastrointestinal disease, prostate cancer and certain inflammatory disorders such as rheumatoid arthritis. If you have risk factors, or aren't sure, it's important to speak with your healthcare provider. BMD tests can tell if you have low bone density and if you need medical treatment. Anyone who has experienced a fracture from an injury that seems minor should be evaluated for osteoporosis.

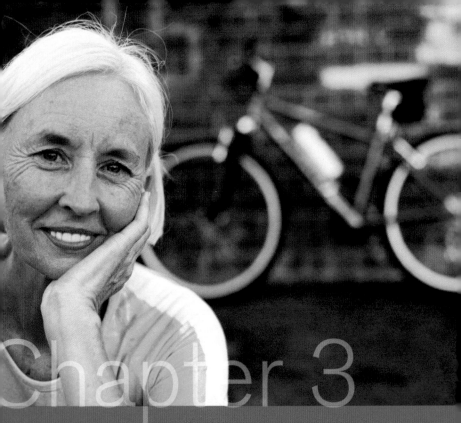

Chapter 3

Detecting Osteoporosis:
The Importance of Testing

Your bones won't tell you if they are becoming weak. They won't creak. They won't ache. In fact, you may have osteoporosis and never know it. For many people, breaking a bone is the first clue that they have osteoporosis. Others can have fractures of the spine and not realize it until they lose height or their spine begins to curve forward. At this point the disease is advanced. In any case, these broken bones can be very painful and lead to long-term problems. More broken bones can follow. That's why it's important to know about the health of your bones—before you break one.

Learning About Your Bone Health

It's important to work with your healthcare provider to find out if you are at risk for osteoporosis.

Diagnosing osteoporosis may involve several steps including:

Medical history. Your healthcare provider will ask you questions to better understand your risk. These questions may concern:

- Medicines you currently take or took in the past
- Other health problems you have currently or had in the past
- Broken bones you've had
- How active you are
- How much calcium and vitamin D you get
- How much alcohol you drink
- Whether you smoke
- If you are a woman, history of menstrual cycle
- Family history of osteoporosis

Physical exam. Your healthcare provider will measure you to see if you have lost any height and check your spine to see if it is curving forward. Either of these could mean that you have had one or more broken bones in the spine.

Tests. Your healthcare provider may order one or more tests, which we will discuss later in this chapter. These include:

- Bone mineral density (BMD) tests, which can measure the amount of bone in different parts of the skeleton
- X-rays or bone scans, which can show other bone problems
- Lab tests, which can give clues about bone loss and new bone formation

BMD Tests

While many tests are used to evaluate bones, the bone mineral density (BMD) test is the only one that can diagnose osteoporosis. A BMD test uses a special machine to measure bone density. In other words, this test lets you know the amount of bone mineral you have in a certain area of bone. A BMD test can tell if you have low bone density before you break a bone. When you repeat the test, it can tell you if your bones are losing density or staying the same. Your BMD, along with your personal risk factors, can predict your chance of having a fracture in the future and can help your healthcare provider decide if you need treatment. If you are being treated for osteoporosis, your healthcare provider may repeat the test every year or two and compare the results to see how

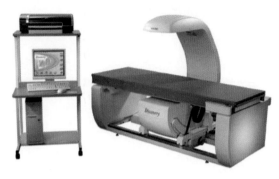

A central DXA (dual energy x-ray absorptiometry) is used to measure bone mineral density.

well your treatment is working.

There are many types of BMD tests. (See Types of BMD Tests, below.) Often, the type of test you have will depend on the equipment available in your community.

Experts recommend a type of BMD test using a central DXA (which stands for dual energy x-ray absorptiometry). They consider it the preferred method to diagnose osteoporosis. Most healthcare providers measure BMD in the hip and/or spine. Breaks in the hip or spine can be the most serious fractures. Sometimes healthcare providers do BMD tests of the wrist, finger or heel. These tests are called peripheral screenings and are not used to diagnose osteoporosis. They can, however, help your healthcare provider decide if a DXA or other tests are needed.

Types of BMD Tests

The methods for measuring bone density include the following:

- DXA (dual energy x-ray absorptiometry)
- pDXA (peripheral dual energy x-ray absorptiometry)
- QUS (quantitative ultrasound)
- QCT (quantitative computed tomography)
- pQCT (peripheral quantitative computed tomography)
- RA (radiographic absorptiometry)
- SXA (single energy x-ray absorptiometry)

Most types of BMD tests, including DXA, use radiation to measure bone density. But for most, the amount of radiation is very small. You would be exposed to 10 to 15 times more radiation flying in a plane roundtrip between New York and San Francisco.

With most of these tests you will remain fully dressed. The test usually takes 5-10 minutes. If you need to have the test again, it is best to have the same type of test at the same place. That allows your healthcare provider to better compare test results. Although it is not always possible to have your BMD test at the same place, it is still important to compare your current BMD test with your last one.

When you have a BMD test your bone density is compared to an "average young

BMD Tests: What the Numbers Mean

The number for your BMD test result is called a T-score. It tells you how your bones compare to those of a healthy young adult's. The difference between your BMD and that of a healthy young adult is described as a "standard deviation" (SD). Usually 1 SD decrease in T-score equals a 10-15-percent drop in bone density. Here's what your T-score means.

If your T-score is . . .	you have. . .
+1 to -1	normal bones
- 1 to -2.5	low bone density or osteopenia
-2.5 or lower	osteoporosis

normal" healthy adult who has reached peak bone density. Test results are expressed in a number called a T-score. The T-score shows how much your bone density is above or below normal when compared to the young normal average person. Your T-score will tell your healthcare provider if you have normal bone density, low bone density (called osteopenia) or osteoporosis. T-scores, however, are not used to diagnose osteoporosis in younger men, premenopausal women and children.

Most experts suggest using Z-scores, rather than T-scores, for younger men and premenopausal women. A Z-score compares a person's BMD to what is expected in another person of the same age and body size. A low Z-score can tell a healthcare provider if a patient should be evaluated for a condition that may be causing bone loss. Z-scores are also used to evaluate BMD in children. A T-score cannot be used in children because they have not yet reached peak bone mass (see page 28).

X-Rays
Healthcare providers do not routinely use standard x-rays for BMD testing. While x-rays can identify broken bones, they are not sensitive enough to detect osteoporosis until 25 to 40 percent of bone density has been lost, and by this time the disease is well advanced.

What Is Osteopenia?

Osteopenia is the medical term for bone density that is lower than normal, but not low enough to be osteoporosis. If you are told that you have osteopenia, it does not always mean you are losing bone or that you will get osteoporosis. Osteopenia is a risk factor for osteoporosis. Now is a good time to make sure you are taking steps to protect your bones. This includes eating a healthy diet, getting regular exercise and talking to your healthcare provider about your bone health.

Do I Need a BMD Test?

Your healthcare provider may recommend a BMD test if you are:
- A postmenopausal woman under age 65 with one or more risk factors for osteoporosis
- A man age 50-69 with one or more risk factors for osteoporosis
- A woman age 65 or older, even without any risk factors
- A man age 70 or older, even without any risk factors
- A woman or man age 50 or older who has broken a bone from an injury that seems minor
- A postmenopausal woman who has stopped taking estrogen therapy (ET) or hormone therapy (HT)
- A man or woman who is being treated for osteoporosis

Some other reasons your healthcare provider may recommend a BMD test include:
- Long-term use of certain medications, including steroids (prednisone and cortisone), some anti-seizure medications, Depo-Provera® and aromatase inhibitors
- A man receiving certain treatments for prostate cancer
- Overactive thyroid gland (hyperthyroidism) or taking high doses of thyroid hormone medication
- Overactive parathyroid gland (hyperparathyroidism)
- X-ray of the spine showing a fracture or bone loss
- Back pain with a possible fracture
- Significant loss of height
- Loss of sex hormones at an early age, including early menopause
- Having a disease that causes bone loss
- Women going through menopause with certain risk factors for breaking a bone

Your healthcare provider may order an x-ray for suspected fractures of the spine or other bones. An x-ray is the most common way to tell if you have a broken bone. People with low BMD can have fractures of the spine that do not cause noticeable pain. It is very important to find these fractures early so that future fractures can be prevented. Over time, these fractures can cause much pain and disability. In addition to x-rays, DXA tests can also be used to look for fractures of the spine. A technique called vertebral fracture assessment (VFA) uses less radiation than a standard x-ray. VFAs can show breaks in the spine and can also show the difference between broken bones and abnormally shaped bones.

Bone Scans
Sometimes healthcare providers order bone scans. A bone scan can tell your healthcare provider if there are changes that may indicate cancer, bone lesions, inflammation or new fractures. These are not the same as bone density tests.

Lab Tests

Lab tests use samples of blood or urine to tell your healthcare provider what is happening in your body. Many people need lab tests to check vitamin D levels. Some of these tests can help your healthcare provider identify conditions that may contribute to bone loss. Other tests may be done called biochemical or bone turnover markers. These tests can provide information about bone loss and formation. They may show if you are losing bone at a faster rate than normal. They may also help your healthcare provider tell if your bones are responding to treatment. Because bone turnover markers do not detect low bone density or diagnose osteoporosis, they cannot take the place of BMD testing.

How to Find a Healthcare Provider

If you are at risk for osteoporosis or already have it, it's important that you have a healthcare provider who knows about the disease. While there is no one type of medical specialty dedicated to osteoporosis, many types of healthcare providers are qualified to diagnose and treat it. Before you make an appointment, ask if a healthcare provider treats patients with osteoporosis.

Also, a healthcare provider who has a background or specialty in "metabolic bone diseases" should be qualified to treat patients with low bone mass or osteoporosis. Here are some examples of healthcare providers who may have experience in osteoporosis prevention, diagnosis and treatment:

- Endocrinologists specialize in disorders related to the glands and hormones.
- Family physicians or general practitioners treat a variety of medical problems in patients of all ages.
- Geriatricians evaluate and treat common conditions and multiple diseases that typically occur among the elderly.
- Gynecologists specialize in the healthcare of women.
- Internists treat a variety of medical problems in adults,

What's Ahead

In the near future, some DXA machines will be able to provide a report that gives information on a person's *Absolute Fracture Risk*. This report incorporates a person's bone mineral density results, age and some of the important risk factors for osteoporosis and fractures. The information in this report will be used to help determine a person's risk of having a fracture in the next 10 years. This prediction of absolute fracture risk will help both healthcare providers and patients decide whether treatment is needed with an osteoporosis medication.

especially conditions that affect the internal organs.

- Orthopedists specialize in the treatment of injuries and disorders of the bones.
- Physiatrists specialize in physical medicine and rehabilitation.
- Rheumatologists specialize in conditions that affect the bones and joints.

Other Healthcare Professionals

Nurse practitioners are registered nurses with advanced education and training who are licensed to treat patients in collaboration with physicians.

Physical therapists with experience in osteoporosis are a resource for patients seeking guidance on appropriate exercise and activities and those to avoid. Physical therapists can perform balance assessment and training that is important in preventing falls and can also help with posture, body mechanics, pain relief and safe movement. A written prescription is usually required to see a physical therapist.

Physician assistants are licensed to treat patients under the supervision of a physician.

Registered dietitians are a resource for nutrition information and special dietary needs. Many hospitals have dietitians on staff.

If you have a primary care physician, ask him or her about osteoporosis. Your own healthcare provider who already knows your overall health may be able to treat you. If you need to see a specialist, your healthcare provider may be able to suggest one for you.

If you don't have a healthcare provider or your healthcare provider can't help you, call your nearest university hospital or community hospital and ask for the department that cares for osteoporosis patients. This department varies from hospital to hospital. For example, in some facilities, the department of endocrinology or metabolic bone disease treats osteoporosis patients, and in others it may be the department of rheumatology, orthopedics or gynecology. Some hospitals have a separate osteoporosis program or women's health clinic that treats osteoporosis patients. Not all hospitals, however, have departments or programs that focus on osteoporosis.

To help you locate a healthcare provider to diagnose or treat your osteoporosis, the National Osteoporosis Foundation (NOF) has developed a Professional Partner's Network (PPN) directory. Any healthcare provider can become a PPN. NOF, therefore, is not able to endorse any of the healthcare providers or healthcare organizations in the PPN directory. For a listing of PPN healthcare providers in your state, visit our NOF Web site at www.nof.org or call (202) 223-2226 or (800) 231-4222 and ask for Patient Education.

Many hospitals now have physician referral services, which may be another way for you to find a healthcare provider who is knowledgeable about osteoporosis. Also check the Web sites of your local hospitals. They usually list the healthcare providers that are on staff, including their sub-specialties and clinical interests. These may include osteoporosis or metabolic bone disease, which includes osteoporosis.

Researching Information

For assistance in researching information, we recommend checking with a librarian at your public library or a medical librarian at your community hospital. Below are websites for information that may be helpful to you.

NOTE: NOF cannot assume responsibility for the quality or trustworthiness of the information found on these Web sites. The content is not necessarily recommended or reviewed by NOF.

For information on clinical trials
www.centerwatch.com   www.clinicaltrials.gov   www.ciscrp.org
For information on clinical study results or to research information from studies
www.pubmed.gov   www.clinicalstudyresults.org
To track new medications in development
www.phrma.org
For drug and supplement information
www.fda.org   www.usp.org
www.pdrhealth.com   www.ods.od.nih.gov
www.drugdigest.org
www.nlm.nih.gov/medlineplus/druginformation.html
For information on laboratory tests
www.labtestsonline.org
For information on complementary and alternative medicine
http://nccam.nih.gov

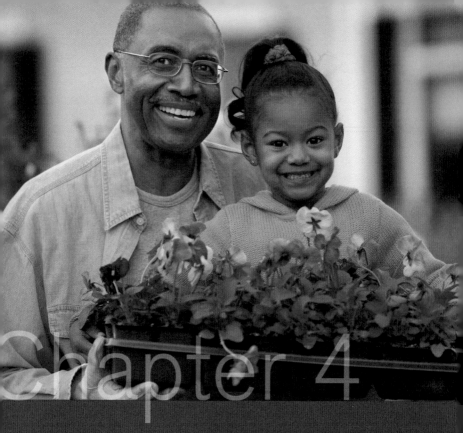

Chapter 4

Treating Osteoporosis

Osteoporosis is a lifelong condition. The progression of the disease varies from person to person and affects some bones more than others. While osteoporosis is not curable, it can be treated and managed. You can help keep bones strong and prevent osteoporosis by exercising, not smoking and getting enough calcium and vitamin D. But these may not always be enough. If you have osteoporosis or low bone density, you should talk to your healthcare provider about whether an osteoporosis medication is right for you.

The Role of Medications

Many osteoporosis medications are now available. If, like many people, you learned you had osteoporosis after breaking a bone, the goal of your treatment will be to recover from your fracture, prevent future fractures and stop bone loss. If you have low bone density and have been fortunate enough to avoid fractures so far, your treatment goal will be to prevent further bone loss and prevent fractures altogether. Many treatments today can help you meet those goals.

For most people, treatment for osteoporosis includes a prescription medication. A number of medications have been approved by the U.S. Food and Drug Administration (FDA) to both prevent and treat osteoporosis. These drugs fall into two main categories: antiresorptives and anabolics. We'll discuss both types below.

Choosing a Treatment

Antiresorptives

Antiresorptive medications slow the breakdown of bone. When you first start taking these medications, you stop losing bone as quickly as you did before, but you should still make new bone at the same pace. Therefore, your bone density may increase slightly. Antiresorptive treatments can prevent further losses in bone mineral density (BMD) and lower your risk of breaking bones.

The antiresorptives available today include:

Bisphosphonates. This is a class of medications that includes alendronate (Fosamax®), ibandronate (Boniva®), risedronate (Actonel®) and zoledronic acid (Reclast®). The FDA has approved these medications for the prevention and/or treatment of osteoporosis in postmenopausal women.

Alendronate and risedronate are also approved to treat osteoporosis in men and to treat steroid-induced osteoporosis. Risedronate is also approved to prevent steroid-induced osteoporosis. Both are available in pill form, and alendronate is also available in a liquid. Alendronate and risedronate increase BMD and reduce the risk of fractures in the spine, hip and other bones.

Ibandronate and zoledronic acid are approved only for women. Ibandronate can be given as a monthly pill. They are also both given by intravenous (IV) infusions, with ibandronate given four times a year and zoledronic acid once a year. Ibandronate increases bone density and reduces the risk of spine fractures. Zoledronic acid increases bone density and reduces the risk of fractures in the spine, hip and other bones.

The more common side effects of bisphosphonates taken by pill include problems with the digestive system such as a burning pain in the chest or esophagus, and pain or trouble with swallowing. Side effects that can occur shortly after receiving an IV bisphosphonate include flu-like symptoms,

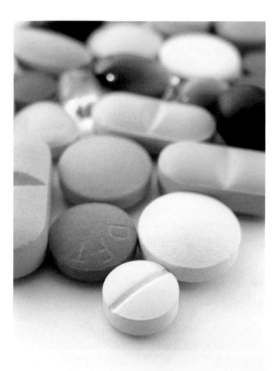 fever, pain in muscles or joints and headaches. Side effects of bisphosphonates taken by pill or IV may include abdominal, bone, joint and muscle pain. There have been rare reports of eye inflammation and very rare reports of death of bone tissue (called osteonecrosis) of the jaw in people who take bisphosphonates either by pill or IV. If you are taking a bisphosphonate, you should let your dentist know before having any dental work. Some invasive dental procedures such as tooth extractions and dental implants could trigger this extremely rare side effect.

Calcitonin. Calcitonin (Fortical®and Miacalcin®) is a synthetic hormone that can slow bone loss and help BMD in the spine. The FDA has approved it only for women who are at least five years past menopause. Calcitonin is available as a nasal spray or injection. The side effects of nasal calcitonin can include nasal irritation, backache, bloody nose and headaches. Possible side effects of injectable calcitonin include nausea, vomiting and flushing. Calcitonin, like any medication, can cause an allergic reaction.

Estrogen therapy (ET) or hormone therapy (HT). These terms refer to estrogen therapy (ET) alone and estrogen with progesterone hormone therapy (HT). These medications are approved for the prevention of osteoporosis in postmenopausal women. They are available under many brand names. Low doses of estrogen can increase BMD and prevent fractures of the spine, hip and other bones. Healthcare providers usually prescribe estrogen with progesterone (HT) because taking estrogen by itself may increase a woman's risk for cancer of the uterine lining (endometrial cancer). A woman who still has her uterus can only take HT. Estrogen therapy (ET) is often prescribed for women who have had hysterectomies.

Although ET and HT are good for bones, large studies have found that they slightly increase the risk of stroke, blood clots and other problems (see page 45). According to the FDA, women should consider other osteoporosis medications before taking ET or HT to prevent osteoporosis. If you decide to take ET or HT, you should take the lowest dose for the shortest period of time. A healthcare provider can help you determine the amount of time that is safest and appropriate for you.

Estrogen agonists/antagonists, also known as selective estrogen receptor modulators (SERMs). These drugs are for women only. They were developed to provide the benefits of estrogen therapy without many of the risks. The only estrogen agonist/antagonist approved so far for osteoporosis is raloxifene (Evista®). Raloxifene increases bone density and reduces the risk of spine fractures. It also reduces the risk of breast cancer in postmenopausal women. Possible side effects include blood clots, swelling, leg cramps and hot flashes.

Anabolics
Anabolic medications speed up your rate of bone formation. Only one anabolic drug, teriparatide (Forteo®), has been approved so far for osteoporosis. It is a type of parathyroid hormone. This medication causes bone growth, increases bone density and reduces the risk of fractures in the spine and other bones. It is indicated for both men and women. It is prescribed for people with very low bone density, people who have had a fracture or those who are at high risk for a fracture. Many people take teriparatide because they had a fracture while taking another osteoporosis medication.

People with certain medical conditions should not take this drug, including those who have hyperparathyroidism, bone or bone marrow cancers, Paget's disease of bone and any other cancers that have spread to the bones. Also, people who have certain abnormal blood test results, including increased calcium levels, should not take this medication. Teriparatide, when given in very high doses for a long period of time, caused a rare bone cancer in rat studies. For this reason, the FDA has approved its use for up to two years only. After stopping teriparatide, bone loss may occur. Most healthcare providers recommend switching to another osteoporosis medication at that time.

Medications Approved to Prevent and/or Treat Osteoporosis

Class and Drug	Brand Name	Form	Frequency
BISPHOSPHONATES			
Alendronate	Fosamax®	Oral (tablet)	Daily/Weekly
Alendronate	Fosamax Plus D™ (2,800 or 5,600 I.U. of vitamin D$_3$)	Oral (tablet)	Weekly
Alendronate	Fosamax®	Oral (liquid solution)	Weekly
Ibandronate	Boniva®	Oral (tablet)	Monthly
Ibandronate	Boniva®	Intravenous (IV)	Four Times per Year
Risedronate	Actonel®	Oral (tablet)	Daily/Weekly/Twice Monthly/Monthly
Risedronate	Actonel® with Calcium	Oral (tablet)	Weekly
Zoledronic Acid	Reclast®	Intravenous (IV)	One Time per Year
CALCITONIN			
Calcitonin	Fortical®	Nasal spray	Daily
Calcitonin	Miacalcin®	Nasal spray	Daily
Calcitonin	Miacalcin®	Injection	Varies
ESTROGEN THERAPY (ET)/HORMONE THERAPY (HT)			
Estrogen*	Multiple Brands	Oral (tablet)	Daily
Estrogen*	Multiple Brands	Transdermal (skin) patch	Twice Weekly/Weekly
ESTROGEN AGONISTS/ANTAGONISTS (ALSO CALLED SERMs)			
Raloxifene	Evista®	Oral (tablet)	Daily
PARATHYROID HORMONE			
Teriparatide	Forteo®	Injection	Daily

Estrogen is also available in various vaginal preparations, in a vaginal ring, as a cream, by injection and as an oral tablet taken sublingually (under the tongue).

The Hormone Debate

Just over a decade ago, estrogen therapy (ET) and estrogen with progesterone hormone therapy (HT) were the only FDA-approved medications to prevent osteoporosis. While estrogen is effective against bone loss in postmenopausal women, it is not appropriate for premenopausal women or for men. The Women's Health Initiative (WHI) study showed that HT was associated with a modest increase in the risk of breast cancer, strokes, heart attacks, blood clots and cognitive (mental) decline.

Follow-up investigation from the WHI showed that women in their 50s, who were closer to menopause, did not have increased risks of heart attacks. Although ET was associated with a similar increase in the risk of strokes, blood clots and cognitive decline, it did not increase the risk of breast cancer or heart attacks.

Because of the results of the WHI study, ET and HT are not used as widely as they once were. Many women still take estrogen to get relief from hot flashes and other menopausal symptoms. If you are one of these women taking estrogen for menopausal symptoms, you are also getting protection from bone loss. But because of the risks, ET and HT should be used in the lowest possible dose for the shortest possible time to meet treatment goals.

If you are considering ET or HT, you should discuss your choices with your healthcare provider to better understand both the possible risks and benefits.

Sometimes healthcare providers prescribe two different osteoporosis drugs at the same time. This may improve bone density more effectively than one drug alone, but experts do not agree about the benefits of combining medications. In fact, there may be some risks of taking two osteoporosis medications, including increased side effects. If your healthcare provider mentions this, you will need to weigh the added cost and consider both the risks and benefits.

Once a medication is approved by the FDA, a healthcare provider can prescribe it. When a healthcare provider prescribes a medication for a different reason than the FDA approved it, this is called prescribing off label. Because the National Osteoporosis Foundation (NOF) takes its guidance from the FDA, NOF is not able to provide information on non-FDA approved treatments for osteoporosis. For example, the safety and effectiveness of alternative therapies to prevent and treat osteoporosis is not currently available.

All medications have a chance of causing side effects, or effects from the drug that you don't want. When you are making a decision about taking a medication, the NOF urges you to discuss your treatment options with your healthcare provider. Together, you can look at both the risks and benefits of taking a medication.

Factors to Consider When Choosing a Treatment

There are many factors to consider when choosing the right osteoporosis treatment for you. A few factors you and your healthcare provider may want to consider are:

Your sex. Calcitonin, estrogen and estrogen agonists/antagonists are approved only for women. Some bisphosphonates and teriparatide are approved for both men and women.

Your age. Some medications may be more appropriate for younger postmenopausal women while some are more appropriate for older women.

If you have not reached menopause. In general, premenopausal women should not take osteoporosis medications. Certain osteoporosis medications are approved for the prevention and treatment of osteoporosis in premenopausal women as a result of the long-term use of steroid medications. In very rare cases, healthcare providers may recommend that some premenopausal women consider taking an osteoporosis medication if they've had a fracture caused by low bone density or have experienced bone loss from a rare medical condition.

How severe your osteoporosis is. Osteoporosis medications work in different ways. A person with more severe bone loss or a broken bone may take a different medication than a person with only minor bone loss.

Other health problems you may have. Your healthcare provider will consider other health problems you have when recommending a medication. If you have had breast cancer or blood clots, for example, you should not take ET or HT. Also, if your bones have been exposed to radiation treatment, you should not take teriparatide.

Personal preference. Do you prefer a pill, liquid or IV medication or one that is given as a nasal spray or an injection? Does it work better for you to take your medication daily, weekly, monthly, several times a year or even once a year? Do you have negative feelings about a particular drug? Any of these factors could influence your treatment decision. It's also important to keep in mind that no two people are the same. How well a medication works or what side effects it will have can vary from one person to the next.

Get the Most From Your Treatment

Many people have trouble taking their medications. People with osteoporosis often take multiple medications for other conditions as well. They may have concerns about the risks and side effects or find the medication instructions complicated. When you have questions about your medications, be sure to speak with your healthcare provider or pharmacist.

When you take an osteoporosis medication, you will not feel your bones getting stronger. This can make it hard to stay on a treatment plan. But it's important that you do so if you want your medication to work. You should take it just as your healthcare provider prescribed it, and you must remember to continue to take it. You also need to exercise regularly and get enough calcium and vitamin D.

If you decide that a treatment is not right for you, don't just stop taking the medication. First, discuss your concerns with your healthcare provider. When prescriptions are not filled, or if they are forgotten, taken incorrectly or stopped early, a person's health condition may not improve or could get worse. Healthcare providers may find it difficult to figure out why a person isn't responding to treatment. They might think the medication did not work or that another health condition may be present. This can lead to extra tests, prescriptions, costs and fractures that could have been prevented by taking the medication as directed.

With antiresorptive medications, the goal of treatment is to prevent further bone loss and to reduce the risk of breaking one or more bones in the future. Your response to treatment is considered good if your bone density either stays the same or improves and if you don't have broken bones. Your healthcare provider may also perform other tests to see if you are responding well to treatment.

With the one anabolic medication, the goal of treatment is to build new bone, increase bone mass, repair tiny defects in bone and reduce the risk of fractures. Your response to this medicine is considered good if both the amount and quality of bone improves and if you have had no broken bones.

To find out how your treatment is working, your healthcare provider will likely repeat the BMD test every one to two years. In some cases, healthcare providers will also use lab tests to see if patients are breaking down bone. While there is no easy way to measure improvement in bone quality, much research is currently underway.

Reporting Adverse Events

No matter how carefully you take your medicines, sometimes they can cause problems. If you have a serious reaction to or problem with a medication, it's important that you or your healthcare provider notify the FDA. You can contact the FDA by calling (800) 332-1088 or by visiting www.fda.gov/medwatch. You may also want to contact the company that made the drug.

How Long to Treat

At this time, healthcare providers don't know for sure how long most osteoporosis drugs stay safe and effective. The one exception is teriparatide (Forteo®). It should be taken for no more than two years. It is not known how long osteoporosis medications stay effective after you stop them. However, research suggests that the benefits of bisphosphonate medications may continue several years or longer after you stop taking them. These drugs stay in the bones for a long time. Not much is known about the safety of taking these medications for longer than 7-10 years. After stopping them, the helpful effects from bisphosphonate medications begin to lessen and bone loss may occur. After stopping an osteoporosis medication, sometimes a different medication is given in order to get the most benefit.

If you have a good response to treatment, your healthcare provider may consider giving you a drug holiday. That means you can stop taking the medicine for a while, but your healthcare provider will continue to monitor your health, bone density, and in some cases, bone breakdown.

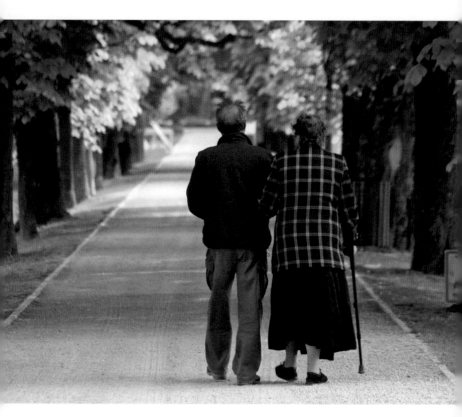

Recovering From Fractures

Even with your best efforts to protect your bones, it's still possible to have a fracture. People most often break a bone in the spine, hip or wrist. But some people break bones in other parts of the body. These can include the ribs, upper arms, pelvis, collarbones, ankles and feet. Regardless of the bone(s) affected, recovery involves more than just healing the bone. Regaining strength and returning to daily activities is an ongoing process. Recovery is a good time to take steps to prevent further bone loss and more broken bones. This includes checking to make sure you are not taking a medication that affects your balance or causes drops in your blood pressure. Both can increase your risk of falling.

Several types of health professionals can help you recover from a fracture. An orthopedic doctor can help repair your broken bone. Physiatrists (doctors who specialize in rehabilitation), physical therapists (PTs) and occupational therapists (OTs) use a variety of methods to help people with osteoporosis function fully after a fracture. Physiatrists often oversee a team of health professionals that may include PTs, OTs and other healthcare professionals to provide well-rounded rehabilitation for the patient. PTs treat pain and discomfort in many ways. These often include exercises to keep the joint moving as well as application of ice and heat. Such treatments are especially important in relieving the muscle spasms and pain that often come with fractures of the spine. In addition, a supervised program of exercises to strengthen the back can help decrease pain and improve function. An OT can teach you techniques that will help you move safely during your daily activities to reduce pain and prevent falls.

Here's what you should know about each of the most common fractures:

Hip Fracture

Hip fractures tend to cause more problems than other broken bones. Most people who break a hip will need surgery to repair it. Some people have problems from the surgery and do not fully recover. Even after surgery, some people have trouble walking again and have to use a wheelchair or walker for a short or long period of time.

If you break a hip, a physiatrist, physical therapist (PT) or occupational therapist (OT) can teach you exercises to help you get better and learn safe ways to move.

Recovery from a hip fracture can take many months. In the early weeks of recovery, your activities will be limited. You may need to rely on others for shopping, cooking, cleaning, bathing and even dressing yourself. Depending on others can be upsetting, especially if you are used to being independent. Remember that this won't last forever—you will get stronger, especially if you are able to walk and do your rehabilitation exercises daily.

The best treatment for hip fractures is to avoid them in the first place. Once you've had one, it's important to take steps to prevent another. Since many hip fractures result from tripping, slipping or loss of balance, you may wish to fall-proof your home (turn to page 60), participate in balance training and learn exercises to increase your muscle strength. The exercises at the end of this book can help you. Check with your healthcare provider about medications you are taking that may cause dizziness, drowsiness or otherwise increase the risk of falling. Also, once you are up and around, have your vision and hearing checked.

Vertebral Fracture

A vertebral fracture is a fracture of one or more bones (vertebrae) of the spine. It can result from a fall, a twisting motion of the torso or from carrying a load that is too heavy for a fragile spine. A movement as simple as rolling over in bed or coughing can cause a vertebral fracture. When this happens, you may feel sharp pain that doesn't get better or you may not feel any

pain at all. When you break more than one vertebra, you may even lose height.

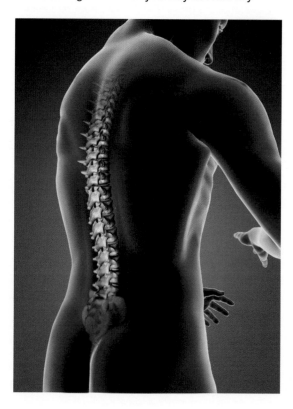

Vertebral fractures can cause your spine to curve forward. This is called kyphosis. It can cause pain as the muscles and other tissues of the back are strained and stretched. The nerves may also become pinched which can cause pain.

If you have a vertebral fracture, it will take several weeks or more to heal. You won't need to have surgery, but you will need to exercise and get rest. During the first week after a fracture, you will need more rest and less activity in order to heal. Soon you will be able to rest less and become more active. This will help you regain strength and mobility. In fact, it's important to increase your activity because too much rest can cause bone loss. Vertebral fractures can sometimes cause other side effects that may need medical treatment. These can include muscle spasms in the back or constipation. No two people recover the same, so listen to your body. Pain and fatigue are signs that you may be pushing yourself too hard.

In some cases, vertebral fractures occur without any noticeable pain. People may learn about these fractures from chest or back x-rays. With all vertebral fractures, you may require an osteoporosis medication to prevent future fractures.

Physiatrists, physical therapists (PTs) and occupational therapists (OTs) can help you learn safe ways to move. They can teach you exercises to help limit your kyphosis. These healthcare professionals can also help you learn to manage your pain. To learn some safe exercises to help your spine, see Chapter 6. For methods to manage pain, see page 57.

Sometimes your healthcare professional may recommend the temporary use of a back brace, jacket or corset to support your spine as you heal from a vertebral fracture. At first you may need to wear it daily while you exercise, when your back is tired or when you have a lot of pain. The support may relieve pain by decreasing movement in the affected area of the spine. It

Surgery for Vertebral Fractures

If you have severe ongoing pain from vertebral fractures, one of these surgeries may help.

VERTEBROPLASTY
This surgery involves injecting bone cement into the fractured vertebral area of the spine. This can reduce pain and make it possible for you to be more active.

KYPHOPLASTY
This surgery is similar to vertebroplasty. It involves first inserting a balloon device into the fractured vertebral area and inflating it to partially restore the height of the vertebra. The space is then filled with bone cement. This can help pain and deformity of the spine due to vertebral fractures.

These procedures are not right for everyone. If you think you might be interested in one of these procedures, you should discuss the possible risks and benefits with your healthcare provider.

will also allow you to return to normal activities sooner and keep kyphosis from getting worse. As your back muscles become stronger, you will use the support less often. It is important not to become too dependent on the spinal support, because using it for too long will keep you from improving muscle and bone strength.

To reduce your risk of vertebral fractures, you may need to avoid some activities or change the ways you do others. For example, you may not be able to pick up your grandchildren or do heavy housework. When carrying groceries, you may need to make several trips with small bags rather than carrying one or two heavy bags (see page 69 for more suggestions).

While surgery for vertebral fractures is often not needed, some surgeries may help relieve pain and restore height to the spine. (To learn more about them, see Surgery for Vertebral Fractures on page 51.)

Wrist Fracture

Wrist fractures are common in people under age 75. Women suffer more wrist fractures around the time of menopause than at any other time. This is probably because of the bone loss that occurs during menopause.

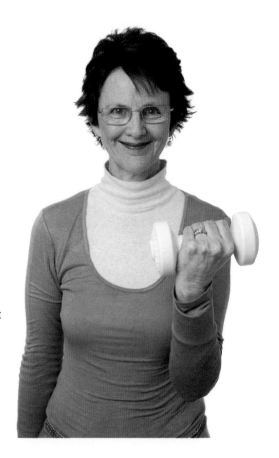

If you are between the ages of 40 and 60, a wrist fracture can be an early warning sign of osteoporosis. When you have a wrist fracture, ask your healthcare provider about getting a BMD test to find out if you have osteoporosis.

While a simple wrist fracture usually heals with a cast or splint, a more complex wrist fracture often requires surgery. If your healthcare provider puts you in a cast or splint, you'll need to wear it for six to eight weeks. During this time, a physiatrist or physical therapist can teach you exercises for your hand, wrist, forearm, elbow and shoulder. Doing these daily will help preserve strength and movement of the wrist, fingers and arm.

After a wrist fracture, you will need help with your daily routine. If the break is in your dominant arm (for example, your right wrist if you are right-handed), you may need help with tasks such as getting dressed, making meals and combing your hair. At the very least, this is frustrating. For people who are frail or have other physical problems, a wrist fracture can be quite disabling.

Beyond Physical Healing

Aside from physical healing, recovery from any type of fracture involves learning to cope emotionally, mentally and spiritually with the changes the fracture may bring. In many cases, a fracture marks the first time you learn you have osteoporosis. In addition to coping with the pain from the fracture and rehabilitation, you also must educate yourself about osteoporosis. There may be necessary, but beneficial, changes in lifestyle and activities that can protect your current bone health.

After a fracture, you may feel that you tire more easily. You may feel depressed, especially when your body image has changed and you fear having more fractures. These challenges may overwhelm you at first. With time and support, however, you can learn to manage them. For more information on dealing with the emotional challenges of osteoporosis, see page 55 in Chapter 5.

To become more active and reduce the effects of osteoporosis on your body and your life, you'll need to find safer ways to do everyday activities. You'll also need to keep up a regular program of exercises to improve your strength, movement and flexibility. The exercises and suggestions at the back of this book can help. But you should never begin any exercise program before speaking with your healthcare provider or other healthcare professional.

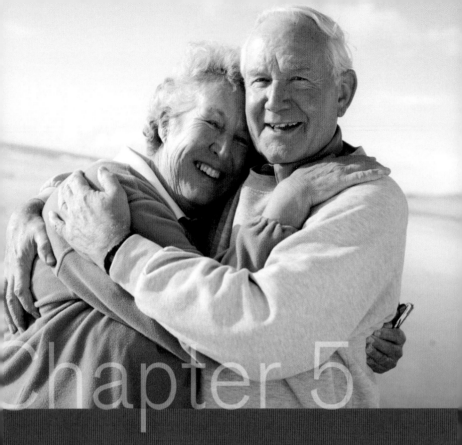

Chapter 5

Living With Osteoporosis

Osteoporosis can affect your life in many ways. Building bones or repairing fractures may not be your only concerns. You may find yourself feeling sad, discouraged or lonely. You may have ongoing pain. If osteoporosis has affected your spine, you may have trouble wearing the clothing styles you prefer. You may be hesitant about doing your favorite activities. You may even be afraid to walk around your own house for fear of falling and breaking a hip or wrist. You may want to learn more about your disease but not know where to look for information you can trust. In this chapter we'll address some of these common concerns.

Finding Support: Building Strength Together®

To help you connect with others who have osteoporosis, the National Osteoporosis Foundation has a program called Building Strength Together®. It provides an opportunity for people to share their concerns, find support and learn more about the disease. You can participate by joining:

- Support groups
- Online community
- Linking Up

Support Groups

Some people with osteoporosis find support groups help them deal with the demands and feelings of living with the disease. Also called self-help groups, support groups bring together people who share common concerns. An osteoporosis support group gives you an opportunity to express feelings and fears. It also allows you to share ideas for coping and learn more about the disease. Understanding that you are not alone can be an important step in coping with osteoporosis. Even if you have family or friends who care for you, sometimes it feels good to talk with someone who also has osteoporosis.

Support group meetings are often held at a local library, hospital, doctor's office, community center or church. Some are organized by people with osteoporosis. Some are sponsored by a hospital or a private medical practice and led by a nurse or other healthcare professional.

To find a support group in your area, you can ask your healthcare provider, local hospital or the National Osteoporosis Foundation (NOF). For general information about NOF support groups or to learn how you or your provider can start a support group:

Visit: www.nof.org

Email: PatientForm@nof.org

Call: (202) 223-2226 or (800) 231-4222

Online Community

NOF's online community brings people together through the Internet to communicate, support each other and learn more about osteoporosis. The online community includes blogs, individual Web pages, discussions, message boards and more. It has rules and structure with moderators to welcome new members, answer questions and enforce rules when necessary. NOF's online community provides privacy by allowing you to control your own personal information.

The benefits of joining an online health community include emotional support, practical information, sense of community, feeling good about helping others and inspiration. People with osteoporosis or osteopenia can participate as well as their family members, caregivers, friends and even healthcare providers. For more information about NOF's online community:

Visit: http://nof.inspire.com

Email: PatientForm@nof.org

Call: (202) 223-2226 or (800) 231-4222

Linking Up
The Linking Up program provides another way for you to contact and even speak with people who have osteoporosis. You have the choice of communicating by postal mail and telephone.

Because women have age-related concerns about menopause and medications, Linking Up for Women is divided into two groups: Linking Up I for Women who are 20-50 years old, and Linking Up II for Women who are 51 and over. NOF also offers Linking Up for Men of all ages. To participate in this program:

Visit: www.nof.org

Email: PatientForm@nof.org

Call: (202) 223-2226 or (800) 231-4222

Coping With Osteoporosis

If your problems seem too big for you to cope with or if you feel depressed for more than two weeks, you should let your healthcare provider know. Your healthcare provider can help you find a health professional that can help you. This may be a psychologist, psychiatrist or social worker.

Making an effort to be active can also help your mood. Even gentle exercise, with your healthcare provider's permission, can give you a boost. A change of scenery can help, too. If you can, get out to shop or meet a friend from time to time. Many people also find it helpful to join a spiritual or religious community, such as a church, synagogue, mosque, or temple.

Getting Your Pain Under Control

For some people, recovery from fractures can be a long and painful process. Sometimes the pain continues even after the fracture heals. Ongoing chronic pain can make it hard to sleep. It can make you depressed or irritable. This, in turn, can make the pain feel worse. Some examples of over-the-counter (OTC) medications that may help with pain relief are aspirin, acetaminophen (Tylenol®), ibuprofen (Advil®, Motrin®) or naproxen (Aleve®). But it is important to remember that these medications can have side effects, especially if you take them at high doses for a long time. Let your healthcare professional and pharmacist know if you take OTC medications. They can help you with stronger pain medicines if you need them. Keep a list of the pain medicines you take and how well they are working.

Medications aren't the only way to manage pain. Some people find that applying cold or heat is helpful. You can use cold in the form of a store-bought cold pack or a bag of frozen peas. As it thaws, the bag of peas will mold to fit the area where you use it. Warm towels and heating pads can also provide relief. Since too much heat or cold can burn or damage the skin, you should not use either one for more than 15 or 20 minutes at a time.

Other ways to help pain include:

Transcutaneous electric nerve stimulation (TENS). This is a method to reduce pain with electrical impulses. A TENS unit is a small box connected by wires to a pair of electrodes. The electrodes are placed on your skin near the site of pain. When the box is switched on, a mild current travels through the electrodes into your body. You may feel tingling or warmth. A treatment lasts from 5 to 15 minutes. You can ask your healthcare provider about getting a prescription for TENS.

Acupuncture. This involves inserting special needles at specific places in the skin. According to ancient Chinese belief, this alters the body's flow of energy into healthier patterns. Acupuncture is gaining acceptance in this country as a way to reduce pain. Your healthcare provider or health insurance company may be able to tell you about acupuncturists in your area. Some health insurance companies offer coverage or discounts for acupuncture.

Biofeedback. This type of therapy uses electronic instruments to measure body functions and then feed that information back to you. A biofeedback specialist uses this information to teach you to control involuntary body responses, such as blood pressure or heart rate. It can also be helpful for managing pain. Your healthcare provider may be able to help you find a biofeedback specialist.

Behavior modification. This is a technique to change habits, behaviors and feelings that can result from ongoing pain. It may include rewards for increasing your physical activity, improving your diet or making other changes in your life.

Physical activity. Being active is a natural way to reduce pain. When you exercise, your body releases substances called endorphins that can relieve pain and boost your mood. Exercise also has many other health benefits. If you have osteoporosis, you should speak with your healthcare professional before you start a new exercise program.

Relaxation techniques. There are several different relaxation techniques that can help people release muscle tension and shift their attention away from pain. Some examples include deep breathing, progressive muscle relaxation and guided imagery. People can learn and practice these and other relaxation techniques from CDs, DVDs/videos, books and classes, as well as trained professionals.

Having Sex—Safely

If you have broken a bone or discover you're at high risk of breaking one, you may be afraid to try certain activities…even sex. That's understandable. But it's possible to have a satisfying sex life with osteoporosis—if you are careful. It's best to avoid positions that cause twisting or forward bending of the spine. Your partner should avoid putting his or her full weight on you. Placing pillows or folded towels under your knees can help keep your spine properly positioned.

The most important thing you can do to have a satisfying relationship is to communicate with your partner. Don't be afraid to try different positions until you find one that is comfortable for both of you. You may also want to speak to a physical therapist (PT) for guidance.

Finding Clothes That Fit and Look Good

Osteoporosis of the spine can lead to changes in the shape of your body. You may get shorter. Your upper back may curve forward and your tummy may protrude. All of these changes can make it hard to find clothes that fit and look good on you. Blouses may be too tight over your back. Collars may gape. Skirts and slacks may ride up under your bust. Skirts and dresses may become too short in the back and too long in the front.

Looking good is closely tied to feeling good about yourself. That's why it is important to find nice-looking clothes that fit well when you have osteoporosis. If you sew your own clothes, you can adapt clothing patterns or store-bought clothes. But if you rely on finding clothes off-the-rack, the following tips will help you find clothing that fits better:

- Overall, wear clothing that is loose, straight or just slightly fitted.

- Look for blouses with jewel, rounded, slight V or soft cowl necklines.

- Choose tops and dresses with dolman or raglan sleeves.

- Add shoulder pads to jackets and blouses to reduce the appearance of sloping shoulders.

- Try dresses with dropped or empire waistlines to hide your tummy.

- Look for jackets and blouses with back yokes or a box pleat in the back. Or try wearing a cape instead of a jacket or coat.

- Use scarves to draw attention to your face and shoulders and away from your back and tummy.

- If you alter your hemlines yourself, look for skirts and dresses with simple straight hems. Avoid difficult pleats or wrapped skirt styles.

- Try different types of bras—long line, front closure, sports-type, or criss-cross straps—to find one that fits well and is comfortable.

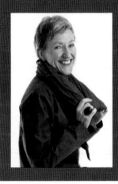

The Magic of Scarves

A simple piece of fabric can become your most useful fashion accessory. By learning a few tricks of folding, twisting or tying, you can add more style to any outfit. Two common shapes for scarves are the square and rectangle, also known as the oblong. The modified ascot is one way you can tie a square scarf. It works best with very soft scarves and looks good with collars and scooped or v-necklines.

Reducing Your Risk of Falls

Each year about one-third of all persons over age 65 will fall. Many of these falls result in a broken bone, often the hip or wrist. Many factors can lead to a fall. They include poor balance, weak muscles, vision problems, certain diseases, alcohol use, certain medications or hazards in the home. Fortunately, there are things you can do to prevent falls. Follow these tips to keep yourself safe.

Fall-Proofing Your Home

FLOORS

- Remove all loose wires, cords and throw rugs.

- Keep floors free of clutter.

- Be sure all carpets and area rugs have skid-proof backing or are tacked to the floor.

- Do not use slippery wax on bare floors.

- Keep furniture in its accustomed place.

BATHROOMS

- Install grab bars on the bathroom walls beside the tub, shower and toilet.

- Use a non-skid rubber mat in the shower or tub.

- If you are unsteady on your feet, you may want to use a plastic chair with a back and non-skid legs in the shower or tub and use a hand-held shower head to bathe.

KITCHEN

- Use non-skid mats or rugs on the floor near the stove and sink.

- Clean up spills as soon as they happen (in the kitchen and anywhere in the home).

BEDROOM

- Place light switches within reach of your bed and a night light between the bedroom and bathroom.

- Get up slowly from sitting or lying since this may cause dizziness.

- Keep a flashlight with fresh batteries beside your bed.

STAIRS

■ Keep stairwells well lit, with light switches at the top and the bottom.

■ Install sturdy handrails on both sides.

■ Mark the top and bottom steps with bright tape.

■ Make sure carpeting is secure.

OUTDOORS

■ Cover porch steps with gritty, weatherproof paint.

■ Install handrails on both sides of porch steps.

AROUND THE HOUSE

■ Place items you use most often within easy reach. This keeps you from having to do a lot of bending and stooping.

■ Use assistive devices to help avoid strain or injury. For example, use a long-handled grasping device to pick up items without bending or reaching. Use a pushcart to move heavy or hot items from the stove or countertop to the table.

■ If you must use a stepstool, use a sturdy one with a handrail and wide steps.

■ If you live alone, you should consider wearing a personal emergency response system (PERS). Also consider buying a portable telephone to take from room to room so you can call for help immediately if you fall.

GOOD ADVICE FOR ANYWHERE

■ If you are unsteady on your feet, use a cane or walker, even if you are going only a short distance.

■ Be careful when you walk on floors that are slippery or that have confusing patterns. You may find these in the lobby of a hotel or bank, a hospital or grocery store.

■ Ask for help or use a cane or walker if you are walking on uneven ground.

■ Slow down. You are more likely to fall if you are in a hurry.

■ Be extra careful when it is wet or icy. During the winter, carry a small bag of sand or kitty litter in your car. If the ground is icy where you park, sprinkle the sand or kitty litter by your car door.

■ Have your vision and hearing checked regularly.

- Talk to your healthcare professional or pharmacist about the side effects of drugs you take. Some can make you feel dizzy.

- Limit alcohol.

- Don't get up too quickly after eating, sitting or lying flat.

- Wear supportive shoes with rubber soles and low heels. Don't walk in socks or slip-on slippers, especially on wood or tile floors.

- Avoid wearing pants and skirts that are too long, spiked heels and tall wedges.

Learning More About Your Disease

You can learn more about osteoporosis by visiting the National Osteoporosis Foundation's Web site, www.nof.org. You can also call NOF toll free at: (800) 223-9994 to request educational materials. NOF has many brochures and publications that can help you learn more about osteoporosis. To learn about becoming a member of NOF, call: (800) 231-4222.

Your healthcare provider can direct you to other good sources of information about osteoporosis.

Notes

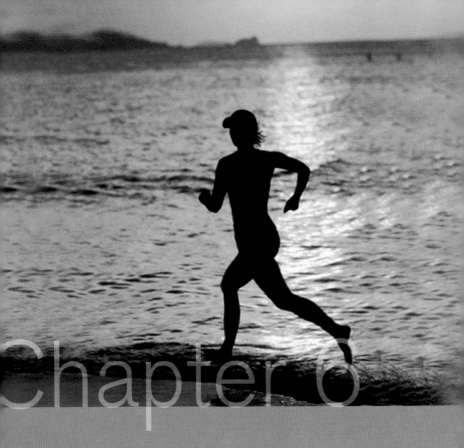

Chapter 6

Safe Movement and Exercises for Daily Living

The first part of this chapter will teach you how to move safely throughout the day. The second part of this chapter contains a series of exercises, including posture exercises, hip and back (spine) strengthening exercises, balance exercises and functional exercises.

Good posture and proper body mechanics are important throughout your life, especially if you have osteoporosis. "Body mechanics" refers to how you move throughout the day.

Safe Movement

Knowing how to move, sit and stand properly can help you stay active while avoiding fractures and disability. Proper posture can also help to limit the amount of kyphosis, or forward curve of the upper back, that can result from vertebral fractures.

One of the most important concepts of body mechanics and posture is alignment. Alignment refers to the relationship of the head, shoulders, spine, hips, knees and ankles to each other. Proper alignment of the body puts less stress on the spine and ensures good posture.

Unsafe Movement

To maintain proper alignment, avoid the following positions or movements:
- Having a slumped, head-forward posture
- Bending forward from the waist
- Twisting of the spine to a point of strain
- Twisting the trunk and bending forward when doing activities such as coughing, sneezing, vacuuming or lifting
- Reaching up for items on high shelves when you could lose your balance and fall

Some exercises can do more harm than good. If you have low bone density, osteoporosis, or slumped posture, you should avoid exercises that involve bending over from the waist, such as:
- Sit-ups
- Abdominal crunches (also referred to as stomach crunches)
- Toe-touches

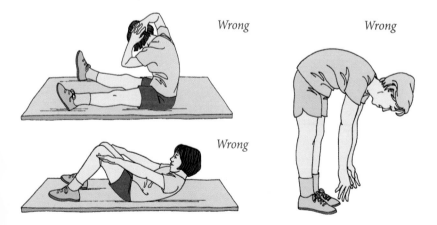

Wrong

Wrong

Wrong

Many exercises and activities such as yoga, Pilates, tennis and golf may need to be avoided or modified because they often involve twisting and bending motions. Bending forward during routine activities also puts stress on the spine and can lead to fractures of the vertebrae.

Sitting

■ When sitting in a chair, try to keep your hips and knees at the same level. Place your feet flat on the floor. Keep a comfortable posture. You should have a natural inward curve to your lower back and a tall, upright upper back.

■ When sitting in bucket seats or soft couches or chairs, use a rolled up towel or pillow to support your lower back.

■ When standing up from a chair, move your hips forward to the front of the chair, and use your leg muscles to lift yourself up.

■ When driving, use the head rest.

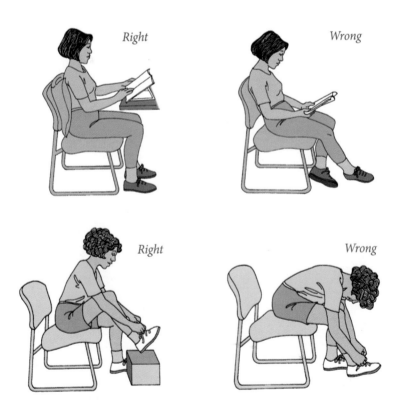

Right   *Wrong*

Right   *Wrong*

- When tying your shoes or drying your feet, sit in a chair. Place one foot on a footstool, box or on your other leg. Lean forward at the hips to tie or dry. Do not bend over or slouch through your upper back. Keep the natural curve of your lower back and a straight upper back.

- When reading, do not lean or slump over. Set your reading material on a desk, table, or on pillows on your lap.

- When sitting at a desk, prop up a clipboard so it slants toward you, like a drafting table.

- Use a footstool or footrest when seated for long periods of time.

- For relief after sitting for a while, do some of the "Bone Healthy Exercises" in the second part of this chapter, such as the Wall Arch or Standing Back Bend (see pages 78 and 79).

Standing

- Keep your head high, chin in, shoulder blades slightly "pinched" together.

- Maintain the natural arch of your lower back as you flatten your abdomen by gently pulling it in.

- Point your feet straight ahead with your knees facing forward.

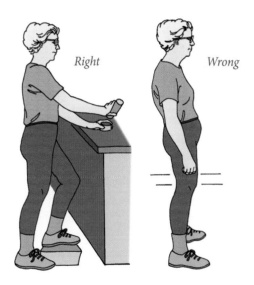

Right   *Wrong*

- While standing in one place for more than a few minutes, put one foot up on a stool or in an open cabinet (if you are in the kitchen). Switch to the other foot every so often. You'll find this much less tiring for your back and legs.

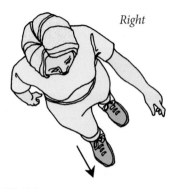
Right

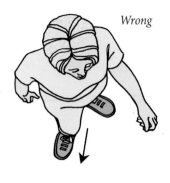
Wrong

Walking

- Keep your head high, chin in, shoulder blades slightly pinched together.

- Keep your feet pointed straight ahead, not to one side (note arrows). Your knees should face forward. Keep your knees slightly bent.

- Avoid letting your knees lock as you bring your weight over your feet.

- Wear secured rubber or other non-slip soles when walking and land lightly on your foot. Don't wear loose slip-on shoes or slippers.

Climbing Stairs

- Use the stairs for exercise and to help with your bone density, but only if your healthcare provider says it's safe for you. Build up gradually with this exercise.

- Keep your head high, chin in, shoulder blades slightly pinched together and abdomen gently pulled in.

- Keep your feet pointed straight ahead, not to one side. Your knees should face forward. Keep your knees slightly bent.

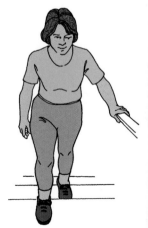

- Instead of putting one foot directly in front of the other, keep your feet a few inches apart, lined up under the hip on the same side.

- For safety, hold the rail while going up and down but try to avoid pulling yourself up by the railing.

- Be especially cautious going downstairs. A fall down the stairs could cause severe injuries.

Bending and Turning

■ Keep your feet flat and about shoulder-width apart from one another.

■ Let both upper arms touch your ribs on the sides, unless you're using one hand for support.

■ As you bend, keep your back upright and straight and your shoulder blades pinched together.

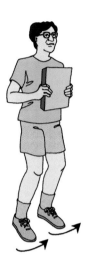

■ Bend only at the knees and hips. Do not bend over at the waist since this will put your upper back into a rounded position which can cause spine fractures.

■ Even when standing to brush your teeth or wash the dishes, try not to bend over at the waist, but rather bend at the knees and hips while keeping your back straight.

■ When changing the direction you're facing, move your feet with your body. Do not twist the spine. Pivot on your heels or toes with your knees slightly bent. Keep nose, knees, and toes pointing in the same direction.

Lifting and Carrying

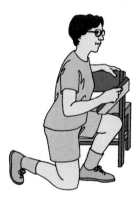

■ Don't lift or carry objects, packages or babies weighing more than 10 pounds. If you are unsure about how much you can lift, check with your healthcare provider, especially a physical therapist.

■ If you are picking up a heavy object, never bend way over so that your back is parallel to the ground. This places a great deal of strain on your back.

■ To lift an object off the floor, first kneel on one knee. Place one hand on a table or stable chair for support if you need it.

- Bring the object close to your body at waist level. Gently pull your abdomen in to support your back and breathe out when you are lifting an object or straightening up. Do not hold your breath. Stand using your leg and thigh muscles.

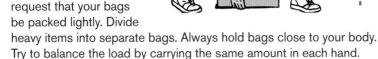

- When carrying groceries, request that your bags be packed lightly. Divide heavy items into separate bags. Always hold bags close to your body. Try to balance the load by carrying the same amount in each hand.

- When unpacking, place bags on a chair or table rather than on a high counter or floor. This prevents unnecessary lifting and twisting of the spine.

- Instead of carrying a heavy pocketbook or purse, consider wearing a fanny pack.

Pushing and Pulling

- When you vacuum, rake, sweep or mop, keep your feet apart with one foot in front of the other. Always face your work directly to keep from twisting your back.

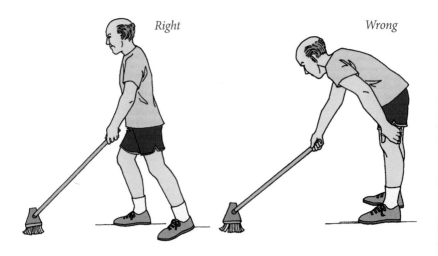

Right   *Wrong*

- Shift your weight from foot-to-foot in a rocking movement. With knees bent and shoulder blades pinched, move forward and back, or from side to side rhythmically.

- Do not bend forward from the waist.

Coughing and Sneezing

- Develop the habit of supporting your back with one hand whenever you cough or sneeze.

- Place your hand behind your back or on your thigh. This protects the spine from damage caused by a sudden bend forward.

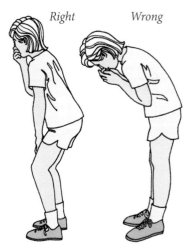

Right *Right* *Wrong*

Getting into Bed

- First, sit down on the side of the bed.

- Lean toward the head of the bed while supporting your body with both hands.

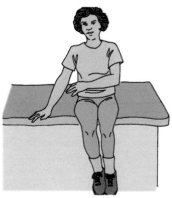

- Then lie down on your side, bringing both feet up onto the bed at the same time.

- Keep your knees bent and arms in front of you. Then roll onto your back in one motion.

- Pull your abdomen in as you roll to support your back and to help prevent twisting.

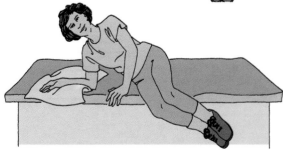

■ Keep nose, knees, and toes pointing in the same direction.

■ Do not lift your head and upper back to move in bed. This puts a great deal of strain on your spine and could cause fractures.

Lying Down and Getting Out of Bed

■ When lying on your side in bed, use one pillow between your knees and one under your head to keep your spine aligned and increase your comfort.

■ When lying on your back in bed, use one or two pillows under your knees and one under your head. Try to avoid using extra pillows to 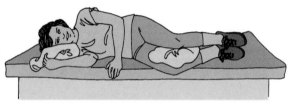 prop your head and upper back since this will put you into a rounded upper back position. But, if you have a rounded upper back posture with a forward head, you may need two pillows to support your neck comfortably.

■ When getting out of bed, reverse the steps you took to get in bed (above):

   1. Keep both arms in front of you.

   2. Pull your abdomen in and breathe as you roll onto your side.

   3. Keep your abdomen pulled in and use your hand to raise your upper body as you carefully place your legs over the side of the bed in one motion.

   4. Sit on the edge of the bed for a moment or two before you stand up.

■ When on your back, never lift your head and upper back to sit up in bed or get out of bed.

Bone Healthy Exercises

The following exercises promote good posture, strength, movement, flexibility and balance in healthy people as well as those with osteoporosis. For more information about exercise, refer to pages 23-26 in Chapter 2. If you have had a fracture recently or if you have very low bone density, you should discuss these exercises with your physical therapist (PT) or healthcare provider before trying them. Remember to avoid all activities that require bending forward from the waist or excessive twisting of the spine.

The following tips and illustrations can help you learn the body parts used in each exercise. These exercises will use many different parts of the body, including the abdomen, pelvis and pelvic floor, trunk and hip flexors.

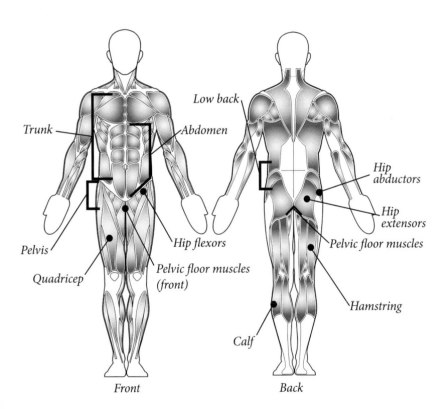

Trunk

Low back

Abdomen

Hip abductors

Hip extensors

Pelvis

Hip flexors

Pelvic floor muscles

Quadricep

Pelvic floor muscles (front)

Hamstring

Calf

Front

Back

Disclaimer: The exercises illustrated in this booklet are intended to aid individuals with low bone density or osteoporosis. You should use this booklet and follow its directions and suggestions only after discussing them with your PT or other healthcare provider.

A little bit of muscle soreness lasting for one to two days after exercise is normal, but none of these exercises should ever hurt in any way while you are doing them or cause soreness for more than one or two days afterwards. If you have pain with any of these exercises or you are not sure if a certain exercise is for you, NOF recommends that you first discuss your concerns with a PT.

How often and how long you exercise and which ones you do depends on your physical ability and exercise goals. Even if you only have ten minutes a day, these exercises can still help you. While all of these exercises are important, you may do some more often than others. For example, if you have good posture but lose your balance or have falls, you may want to do each posture exercise one or two times per week, but spend several minutes each day on the balance exercises. If you struggle to stand up from a chair or climb stairs, you may want to do each of the key functional exercises every day.

These exercises are designed to be done along with a weight-bearing exercise program. Therefore, these exercises do not replace the need for walking or doing other weight-bearing activities (see page 26 for information on weight-bearing exercises).

For exercises that involve lying on the floor, you may want to place a blanket or thick mat under you for comfort. If you cannot get up and down from the floor, you may do them on a firm bed.

The exercises in this chapter are divided into four sections:

■ Posture Exercises

■ Hip and Back (Spine) Strengthening Exercises

■ Balance Exercises

■ Functional Exercises

Each section begins with a list of the key exercises for your program. After this list are additional exercises that are also important. Some exercises fit into more than one section. For example, some of the hip strengthening exercises are very helpful for good balance. For the greatest benefit, you should include all of the exercises listed in the section you are working on.

You can improve your posture with the following stretching and strengthening exercises.

POSTURE EXERCISES

KEY EXERCISES				
01	Pelvic Lift Exercise	07	Wall Arch Stretch
02	Basic Abdominal Exercise	08	Corner Stretch
03	Basic Abdominal with Leg Slide	09	Standing Back Bend
04	Basic Abdominal with Arm Raise	10	Standing Calf Stretch
05	Chin Pulls/Neck Lengthening	11	Quadriceps & Hip Stretch
06	Upper Back Strengthening	12	Sitting Hamstring & Calf Stretches

RELATED EXERCISES		
18	Prone Leg Lifts
19	Prone Trunk Lifts

01 Pelvic Lift Exercise

The pelvic floor muscles are the muscles that control the flow of urine (refer to the illustration on page 73 to see where the pelvic floor muscles are located).

■ While lying down, sitting or standing, think of pulling your pelvic floor muscles up as if to prevent urine flow.

■ Hold for a count of 5-10 seconds.

■ Let go gradually.

■ Repeat 5-10 times, 2-4 times per day.

Start by performing this exercise while lying down, then progress to sitting and standing.*

*To control leakage of urine during coughing, sneezing and strenuous movements, perform exercise by pulling up and releasing 10 times quickly. Do this 2-4 times per day.

Benefit: Helps prevent incontinence (being unable to control leakage of urine) and prolapsed (dropped or fallen) uterus or bladder. Provides support for lower back and trunk.

02 | Basic Abdominal Exercise

■ Lie on your back with knees bent and feet flat on the floor with a small pillow under your head.

■ You will have a little space between the floor and the arch of your low back.

■ Tighten your abdominal muscles by pulling your abdomen in.

■ Think about pulling your navel in toward your spine. Try to keep the space between the floor and the arch of your low back.

■ Hold for 2 seconds.

■ Relax. Repeat 10 times, once each day. When you can do this without much effort, replace it with exercises #3 and #4 below.

Benefit: Strengthens and flattens abdominal muscles.

03 | Basic Abdominal Exercise with Leg Slide

■ Perform the abdominal pull-in exercise.

■ Slide one leg out as far as you can, keeping your abdomen pulled in.

■ Return to the original position while keeping your abdomen pulled in.

■ Relax. Repeat 5 times with each leg, once each day.

Benefit: Strengthens and flattens abdominal muscles and stretches the muscles on the front of the hip.

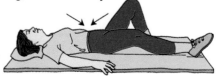

04 | Basic Abdominal Exercise with Arm Raise

■ Perform the abdominal pull-in exercise.

■ Keeping your abdominal muscles pulled in, bring one arm up over your head with your elbow straight, while squeezing your shoulder blades in, and then return it to your side.

■ Be sure to keep your abdomen tight and your back in the starting position without letting it rise off of the floor as you move your arm.

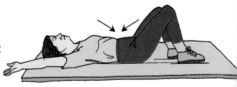

■ Relax.

■ Repeat 5 times with each arm, once each day.

Once you can do this without your back lifting off the floor, you can do both arms at the same time.

Benefit: Strengthens and flattens abdominal muscles and stretches chest muscles.

For proper posture, you need a strong trunk. You should start by strengthening your pelvic floor and abdominal muscles to create a solid core. All other exercises should start with a pelvic lift and an abdominal pull-in.

05	Chin Pulls/Neck Lengthening

■ In a seated position, pull your chin in, as if you could move it to the back of your neck.

■ Look straight forward, not up or down.

■ Keep your head high, lengthening the back of your neck.

■ You will feel a stretch in the back of your neck and a flattening of your upper back.

■ Push your hands down on your thighs to help your back become as straight as possible.

■ Hold 2 seconds.

■ Repeat 10 times, once each day.

Benefit: Corrects forward head posture.

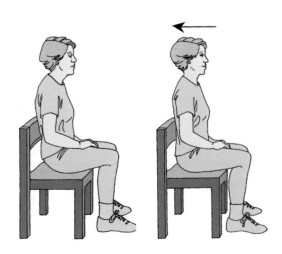

06 Upper Back Strengthening

■ Sit or stand as tall as you can with your chin in (as in Chin Pulls exercise).

■ Keep abdomen pulled in, chest gently lifted and both feet flat on the floor.

■ Place arms in a "W" position with your shoulders relaxed, not hunched.

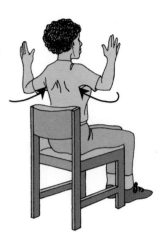

■ Bring your elbows back, pinching shoulder blades together.

■ Hold for a slow count of 1-2-3.

■ Relax for a slow count of 1-2-3.

■ Repeat 10 times, once each day.

Benefit: Decreases forward tilt of the head and rounded shoulders. Flattens and strengthens upper back and abdomen.

07 Wall Arch Stretch

■ Face a wall with your feet six inches from the wall and six inches apart from each other.

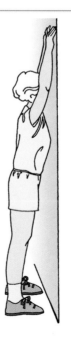
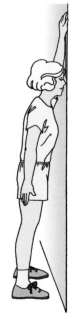

■ Take a deep breath and stretch your arms up to touch the wall.

■ Try to keep your abdomen pulled in.

■ Hold 10 seconds, lower your arms.

■ If this strains your shoulders, you may need to start by lifting one arm at a time.

■ Repeat 3-5 times, 3 times per week.

Benefit: Flattens upper back. Strengthens abdomen and stretches shoulders.

08 | Corner Stretch

■ Stand in the corner of a room with your arms extended to the walls at shoulder level.

■ Step one foot forward, letting that knee bend.

■ Lean onto the front leg, bringing your head and chest toward the corner.

■ Hold for 20-30 seconds.

■ Stand up straight and switch feet.

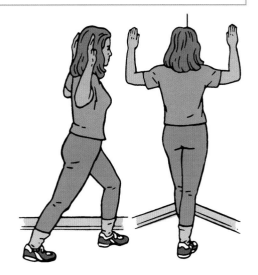

■ Repeat it on the other side.

■ Do 2 on each side, 3 times per week.

Benefit: Stretches shoulders, flattens upper back. Improves rounded shoulders.

09 | Standing Back Bend

Keep your abdominal muscles pulled in during each stretch. If you have balance problems, stand with your back next to a counter or in front of a wall.

Level 1

■ Make two fists and place them on your lower back below your waist.

■ Arch backwards slowly, while taking a deep breath.

■ Relax and repeat 5-10 times.

■ Do once each day.

Level 2

■ When you can do Level 1 comfortably, progress to placing your fists on your middle back at waist level.

■ Relax and repeat 5-10 times.

■ Do once each day.

Level 3

■ When you can do Level 2 comfortably, progress to placing your fists higher up on your back above waist level, if possible.

■ Repeat 10 times, once each day.

Benefit: Restores healthy lower back curve. Decreases rounded upper back.

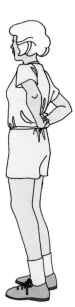

10	Standing Calf Stretch

Starting position for both leg stretching exercises:
Reach out to hold a counter or the back of a chair. Stand with your feet pointing ahead and hip width apart. Keep your knees relaxed and lined up over your second toe. Hold your abdomen flat, back straight and shoulder blades gently pinched together.

■ From starting position (above), step one foot forward, keeping your back foot flat on the floor with your leg straight.

■ Keep your toes and knees facing forward.

■ Keep your body straight and abdomen gently pulled in.

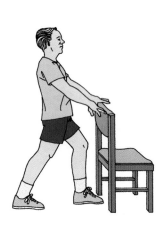

■ Lean weight forward as you bend the front knee to stretch the calf of the back leg.

■ Hold for 30-60 seconds.

■ Repeat with the other leg.

■ Do 2 on each leg, 3 times per week.

11 | Quadriceps & Hip Stretch

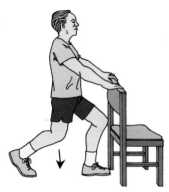

■ Start with calf stretch position.

■ Lift up your heel and bend the knee of the leg behind you.

■ Lean weight forward on bent front knee and push back knee down as if reaching it to the floor for the stretch.

■ Hold 20-30 seconds.

■ Repeat with the other leg.

■ Do 2 on each leg, 3 times per week.

Benefit: Stretches calf and thigh muscles and front of hip. Increases weight-bearing through the hip. Improves balance and standing posture.

12 | Sitting Hamstring & Calf Stretches

■ Sit with your back straight, abdomen pulled in and arms resting at your sides or on your thighs.

■ Slowly straighten your knee, keeping your back very straight (don't slump and let your back round out).

■ After your knee is as straight as possible, bend your ankle so that your foot points upward toward the ceiling or back toward your knee (stretches your calf).

■ Hold 10 seconds.

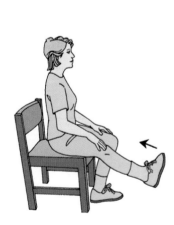

■ Relax and lower your leg to the starting position.

■ Repeat the sequence with the other leg.

■ Do 3-5 on each leg, 3 times per week.

Benefit: Stretches calf muscles (back of lower leg) and hamstrings (back of thigh). Improves posture.

HIP AND BACK (SPINE) STRENGTHENING EXERCISES

KEY EXERCISES				
	13	Hip Flexor Strengthening	17	Sidelying Knee Lifts
	14	Hip Abductor Strengthening	18	Prone Leg Lifts
	15	Hip Extensor Strengthening	19	Prone Trunk Lifts
	16	The Bridge		

RELATED EXERCISES				
	22	Wall Slide	24	Chair Rises
	23	Wall Sit	06	Upper Back Strengthening

The following exercises strengthen the muscles around the hip and along the spine to help decrease the risk of a fracture in these areas. They can also help your balance to decrease the risk of a fall.

For the following strengthening exercises, do the pelvic lift and abdominal pull-in during the entire exercise. If you can do the exercise without your muscles being tired, you should add weight to make it more difficult. Once the weight becomes easy, you should increase it.

13 Hip Flexor Strengthening

■ Stand beside a chair, standing as tall as possible.

■ Lift your knee up as if marching.

■ Do not lift it higher than your hip.

■ Lower and repeat 10 times.

■ Repeat with the other leg.

■ Do this 2-3 times per week.

■ If you can, add an ankle weight that is heavy enough that you cannot lift it more than 10 times.

Benefit: Strengthens the hips. Improves balance.

14 Hip Abductor Strengthening

- Stand straight and hold onto the back of a chair, without bending at the waist or knee.

- Place other hand on the top of your pelvis and raise this leg straight out to the side.

- Make sure that the toes point forward and your pelvis (and hand) don't rise up.

- Lower the leg and repeat 10 times.

- Change sides and repeat the exercise with the other leg.

- Do this 2-3 times per week.

- If you can, add an ankle weight that is heavy enough that you cannot lift it more than 10 times.

Benefit: Strengthens the hips. Improves balance.

15 Hip Extensor Strengthening

- Stand straight and hold onto the back of a chair.

- Bend forward about 45 degrees at the hips.

- Lift one leg straight out behind you as high as possible without bending your knee or moving your upper body.

- Lower leg and repeat 10 times.

- Change sides and repeat the exercise with the other leg.

- Do this 2-3 times per week.

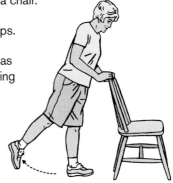

If you can, add an ankle weight that is heavy enough that you can not lift it more than 10 times.

Benefit: Strengthens the hips. Improves balance.

16 The Bridge

■ Lie on your back with knees bent and feet flat.

■ Keep your arms at your sides.

■ Press your head and shoulders down.

■ Lift your buttocks up so your body raises from the floor.

■ Lower, relax and repeat 10 times.

■ When you can do this 10 times without difficulty, do this exercise with one leg out flat, lifting body with the other leg.

■ Do 10 on one side and then 10 on the other.

■ Do this exercise 2-3 times per week.

Benefit: Strengthens hips. Improves balance.

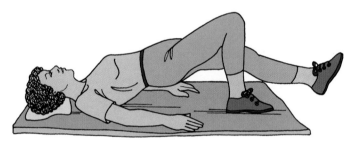

17 Sidelying Knee Lifts

■ Lie on your side with knees bent, pelvis forward and abdomen gently pulled in.

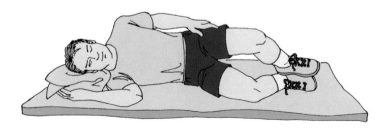

- Lift the top knee, keeping feet together.

- Do 10 on one side and then 10 on the other.

- Do this exercise 2-3 times per week.

Benefit: Strengthens hip and abdominal muscles.

18 Prone Leg Lifts

- Lie on your abdomen with hands at your sides.

- Place a towel under your forehead and your shoulders and towel or pillow under your abdomen for comfort (see illustration).

- Bend your right leg slightly and lift your thigh off the floor.

- Keep your foot relaxed.

- Lower and repeat 10 times.

- Then do 10 on the other side.

- Do this 2-3 times per week.

- If you can, add an ankle weight that is heavy enough that you cannot lift it more than 10 times.

- If this causes back pain, try adding another pillow under your abdomen or replace this exercise with the Hip Extensor strengthening exercise.

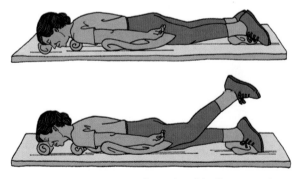

Benefit: Strengthens lower back and buttocks. Stretches hip flexors and the front of the thighs.

- Lie on your stomach as described in Prone Leg Lifts exercise above.

- Place a towel under your forehead and a pillow under your abdomen for comfort (see illustration).

- Keep your abdomen pulled in, feet down, and head in a normal position.

- With hands at your sides, lift your upper back while pinching shoulder blades together.

- Hold for 1 to 3 seconds.

- Relax and repeat.

- Inhale going up and exhale going down.

- Do not arch your neck up.

- Do 10 times, once each day.

Benefit: Strengthens back.

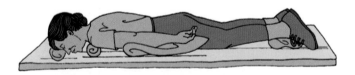

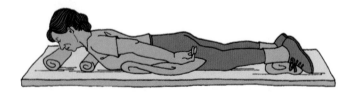

BALANCE EXERCISES

KEY EXERCISES		
	20	Balance Training Progression
	21	Toe Raises/Heel Raises

RELATED EXERCISES				
	10	Standing Calf Stretch	18	Prone Leg Lifts
	13	Hip Flexor Strengthening	19	Prone Trunk Lift
	14	Hip Abductor Strengthening	22	Wall Slide
	15	Hip Extensor Strengthening	23	Wall Sit
	16	The Bridge	24	Chair Rises
	17	Sidelying Knee Lifts		

You can improve your balance with the following exercises which can decrease your risk of a fall and fracture. These exercises are especially important if you have fallen one or more times in the past year or if you lose your balance as you do normal activities.

Leg strengthening exercises will help balance. Hip strengthening exercises can be included in your balance training exercise program.

When you do balance training exercises, you should feel a little wobbly in your legs and feet, but you should not feel like you could fall. The goal of these exercises is to hold the position for 20-30 seconds and progress to the next level when you no longer wobble.

When you are first doing an exercise, you may need to hold onto a stable chair or table with both hands. When you no longer wobble, hold on with one hand only. Then progress to touching the chair or table with one fingertip only. As you become steadier, hold both hands two inches above the chair or table. When you can do this without wobbling, keep your hands two inches above the chair or table and do the exercise with your eyes closed.

To make each exercise harder, stand on a soft surface, such as a pillow. Do the exercises on each leg. Balance exercises can be done every day.

20 | Balance Training Progression

- Stand with feet tight next to each other.

- Stand with one foot in front of the other with the front heel touching the back foot's big toe.

- Stand with one foot in front of the other like you are on a tight rope.

- Stand on one leg only.

Benefit: Improves balance. Prevents falls.

21 | Toe Raises/Heel Raises

- Stand straight and hold onto the back of a chair, without bending at the waist or knees.

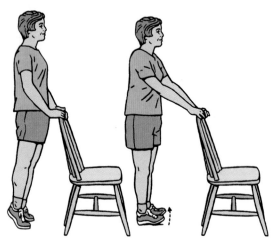

- Rise up on your toes and then back onto your heels. When you rise up onto your toes, imagine you are moving your head up to the ceiling.

- Repeat 10 times.

- Hold on to the chair as little as possible to challenge your balance.

- Do this once each day.

Benefit: Strengthens lower legs. Helps balance.

FUNCTIONAL EXERCISES

KEY EXERCISES	22	Wall Slide		24	Chair Rises
	23	Wall Sit			

RELATED EXERCISES	01	Pelvic Lift Exercise		10	Standing Calf Stretch
	02	Basic Abdominal Exercise		13	Hip Flexor Strengthening
	07	Wall Arch Stretch		21	Toe Raises/Heel Raises

Doing exercises that are similar to everyday activities will keep you strong in these activities. Some of these exercises can also help your balance to decrease the risk of a fall.

Starting position for wall sit/wall slide:

■ Stand with your heels one shoe-length from the wall.

■ Keep your feet straight ahead and shoulder width apart.

■ Place your buttocks, palms of your hands and shoulders against the wall.

■ Tuck your chin in so that the back of your head is as close to the wall as possible. Pull in your abdomen the entire time.

22 Wall Slide

■ Begin with starting position for wall sit/wall slide.

■ Slide up and down, bending your knees half-way to a sitting position.

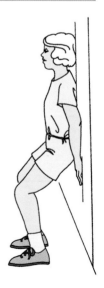

■ Keep your shoulders back and abdomen flat.

■ Keep your back flat.

■ Do this 10 times, 2-3 times per week.

Benefit: Strengthens thighs, abdomen, and back. Decreases rounded upper back and forward head posture. Improves leg alignment.

23 Wall Sit

- Begin with starting position for wall sit/wall slide.

- To increase thigh strength and place positive stress on the hip, place your feet 1 to 1½ shoe lengths from the wall and slide down the wall. Hold the "wall sit" for up to 30 seconds.

- Keep your knees lined up over your second toe.

- Repeat 2 times, 2-3 times per week.

Benefit: Strengthens thighs, abdomen, and back. Decreases rounded upper back and forward head posture. Improves leg alignment.

24 Chair Rises

- Sit on the front edge of a chair and rise to a standing position and gently sit back down without using your arms. It may be helpful to cross your arms on your chest to prevent using them.

- Keep your knees and feet hip width apart at all times.

- Use the strength of your legs to stand and sit.

- If you are not able to do this without using your arms, place a pillow on the chair.

- The goal is to stand and sit 10 times in a row. Once you can complete the set of 10, move the exercise to a lower chair to make it harder.

- Do this exercise once each day.

Benefit: Strengthens legs. Helps with safety when getting up from a chair to stand.

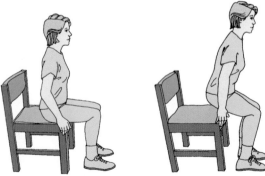

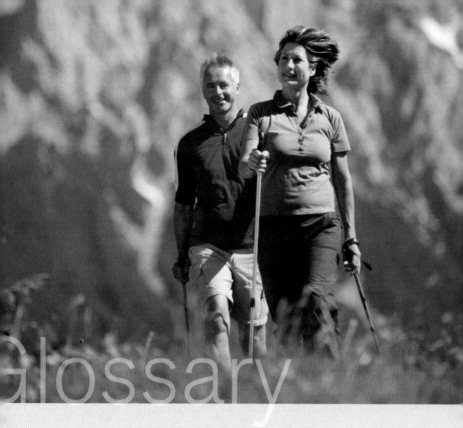

Glossary

Glossary of Commonly Used Terms

Actonel®–See risedronate.

Alendronate–A medication that can prevent and treat osteoporosis in women and men. It is in a class of medications called bisphosphonates. It is taken as an oral tablet once weekly or daily. The brand name is Fosamax®.

Anabolic medications–A category of medications that help build bone. At this time, teriparatide is the only anabolic osteoporosis medication.

Antiresorptive medications–A category of medications that slow the breakdown of bone. These medications protect bone mineral density and reduce the risk of fractures. Most osteoporosis medications are antiresorptive medications. These medications include bisphosphonates, calcitonin, estrogen therapy/hormone therapy and an estrogen agonist/antagonist which is also called a selective estrogen receptor modulator (SERM).

Balance exercises–Exercises that strengthen your legs and challenge your balance, such as Tai Chi. Balance exercises can decrease your risk of falls.

Bisphosphonate medications–A class of antiresorptive medications that slow the breakdown of bone. They include alendronate, ibandronate, risedronate and zoledronic acid.

Bone density–See bone mineral density (BMD).

Bone mass–The amount of mineral content in your bones. Bone mass is not corrected for bone size.

Bone mineral density (BMD)–Average concentration of minerals in your bones. BMD is corrected for bone size and is also called bone density.

Bone mineral density (BMD) test–A test that uses a special machine to measure bone density. Some people also call it a bone mass measurement test or bone density test. It helps doctors find out if your bones are becoming weak and if you are likely to have a fracture.

Boniva®–See ibandronate.

Calcitonin–A medication to treat osteoporosis in women at least five years past menopause. It is a hormone that helps regulate how your body uses calcium. Calcitonin is available as a nasal spray (brand names are Fortical® and Miacalcin®) or injection (brand name is Miacalcin®) to treat osteoporosis.

Calcium–A mineral needed to build strong bones. For bone health, it is important to eat foods rich in calcium, such as milk, dairy products, fortified foods and other calcium rich foods. If you do not get enough calcium through your diet, it is important to take a calcium supplement.

Calcium citrate–A type of calcium supplement. Calcium supplements from calcium citrate do not need to be taken with food for absorption.

Calcium carbonate–A type of calcium supplement. Calcium carbonate should be taken with food for best absorption.

Collagen–A major component of bone. Collagen is a protein that gives bones a flexible framework.

Corticosteroids–Medications that relieve inflammation and are much like certain hormones made by your own body. If you take them for long or at high doses, they can cause bone loss that leads to osteoporosis and fractures. These medications are also known as steroids and glucocorticoids. They are used to treat many conditions such as arthritis and asthma.

Daily value (DV)–The Food and Drug Administration (FDA) lists DVs on the "Nutrition Facts" panel of foods to help consumers determine the amount of nutrients in each product. DVs can help people decide if a food is a good source of certain nutrients, such as calcium and vitamin D.

Dual-energy x-ray absorptiometry (DXA)–A test to detect low bone density and diagnose osteoporosis. Most experts consider it the preferred method to diagnose osteoporosis. This test can be performed on the spine, hip, forearm, heel or total body.

Endocrinologist–A physician who treats the endocrine system, which includes the glands and hormones that help control the body's metabolic activity. In addition to osteoporosis, conditions often treated by endocrinologists include diabetes, thyroid disorders and pituitary diseases.

Estrogen–A female hormone that controls sexual development and the menstrual cycle. It also plays an important role in maintaining healthy, strong bones in women. The body produces very little estrogen after menopause.

Estrogen agonist/antagonist–A type of medication that is also called a selective estrogen receptor modulator (SERM). It was developed to provide the benefits of estrogen therapy without some of the risks. This type of medication is for women only. The only estrogen agonist/antagonist that is currently approved for osteoporosis is raloxifene (Evista®).

Estrogen therapy (ET)/hormone therapy (HT)–These terms refer to estrogen therapy (ET) alone and estrogen with progesterone hormone therapy (HT). While these medications can prevent osteoporosis in postmenopausal women they also increase the risk of other health problems. A woman who still has her uterus can only take HT. ET/HT are available under many brand names.

Evista®–See raloxifene.

Family physician–A physician with a broad range of training that includes surgery, internal medicine, obstetrics and gynecology and pediatrics. Family physicians place special emphasis on caring for an individual or family on a long-term, continuing basis.

Forteo®–See teriparatide.

Fosamax®–See alendronate.

Fracture–A broken bone. A fracture is often the first sign of osteoporosis. While the most common osteoporosis fractures occur in the hip, vertebrae (bones in the spine) and wrist, these fractures also occur in many other bones.

Functional exercises–Exercises that improve how well you move and help you in everyday activities to decrease your risk of falls and fractures.

Geriatrician–A family healthcare provider or internist who specializes in treating patients age 65 and older. This type of physician receives additional training on the aging process and is able to evaluate and treat common conditions and multiple diseases that typically occur among the elderly.

Glucocorticoids–See corticosteroids.

Gynecologist–A physician who diagnoses and treats conditions of the female reproductive system and associated disorders. A gynecologist may serve as primary healthcare provider for women and follow a patient's reproductive health over time.

Healthcare provider–A person who is trained and licensed to provide healthcare services. Healthcare providers include medical doctors, nurse practitioners, physician assistants, physical therapists and other health professionals.

Hormone therapy–See Estrogen therapy (ET)/hormone therapy (HT).

Ibandronate–A medication that can prevent and treat osteoporosis in women. It is in a class of medications called bisphosphonates. Ibandronate can be taken as an oral tablet once monthly or given by intravenous (IV) infusion every three months. The brand name is Boniva®.

Idiopathic juvenile osteoporosis–This condition affects children between the ages of 1 and 13. Its cause is unknown. Children with this condition tend to have fractures, particularly of the legs and spine. Fortunately, this type of osteoporosis usually goes away at adolescence.

Internist–A physician who is trained in the essentials of overall care of general internal medicine in adults. An internist diagnoses and nonsurgically treats many diseases of the body. An internist also provides long-term comprehensive care in the hospital and office.

Kyphoplasty–A treatment for severely painful fractures of the vertebrae (bones in the spine). It involves inserting a balloon device into a fractured vertebra and inflating it to restore the height of the vertebra. The space is then filled with bone cement. This can help pain and possibly deformity of the spine due to recent fractures of the vertebrae.

Kyphosis–Abnormal forward curving of the spine caused by fractures of the vertebrae.

Medications–Substances or combinations of substances that are primarily used or given to treat or prevent disease. Osteoporosis medications fall into two categories: 1) antiresorptive medications; and 2) anabolic medications. Medications are also called medicines or drugs.

Menopause–The time in a woman's life when she stops having menstrual periods and her estrogen levels drop. This can happen naturally or when the ovaries are removed surgically. For many women, bone density decreases quickly in the first few years after menopause.

Nurse practitioner–A registered nurse with advanced education and training who is licensed to treat patients in collaboration with physicians.

Occupational therapist (OT)–A healthcare professional who can help you recover from a fracture. An OT can teach techniques that will help you move safely during your daily activities to reduce pain and prevent falls.

Orthopedist–A physician who treats injuries and disorders of the musculoskeletal system. This system includes bones, joints, muscles and tendons. An orthopedic surgeon operates to correct, fix or replace joints and limbs. Alternate spelling for orthopedic is orthopaedic.

Osteoarthritis–The most common form of arthritis–sometimes called "wear and tear"–is a disease of joint cartilage. Cartilage is the tough tissue that covers the ends of the bones where they meet to form joints. When joint cartilage breaks down, the bones can rub against each other. Bone spurs often form and the joints become stiff and painful. Aside from its name, osteoarthritis has little in common with osteoporosis.

Osteopenia–Low bone mass. This means bone mass or bone mineral density is lower than normal, but not yet low enough to be considered osteoporosis. A person in this category may benefit from taking an osteoporosis medication depending on his or her risk factors for osteoporosis and fractures.

Osteoporosis–A condition in which the bones become so porous and weak that they are likely to break from a minor injury. A person with osteoporosis can break a bone from a minor fall, picking up a bag of groceries, and in more serious cases, from a simple action such as a sneeze. While the most common osteoporosis fractures occur in the hip, vertebrae (bones in the spine) and wrist, these fractures also occur in many other bones.

Ovaries–The two glands that produce eggs and sex hormones in women. When the ovaries stop producing estrogen at menopause or are removed surgically, bone loss can occur rapidly.

Parathyroid hormone–A hormone made by the four parathyroid glands that are close to the thyroid gland in the neck. Its main job is to control the amount of calcium in the blood.

Peripheral DXA–A test of bone density in bones other than the hip or spine. This type of test is often done on the wrist, finger and heel.

Peak bone mass–The point at which you have the most bone you will ever have. This usually is between the ages of 18-25.

Physiatrist–A doctor who specializes in rehabilitation. A physiatrist can help you recover from a fracture, regain function and reduce pain. Physiatrists often oversee a team of health professionals that may include PTs, OTs and other healthcare professionals to provide well-rounded rehabilitation for the patient.

Physical therapist (PT)–A healthcare professional who can help you after a fracture. PTs treat pain and discomfort with exercises to keep the body moving. They also use ice, heat and other treatments to help a person recover after a fracture. A PT can also help you learn an exercise program to help ease pain, make you stronger and better able to perform your daily activities as well as to prevent fractures.

Physician assistant–A healthcare professional who is licensed to treat patients under the supervision of a physician.

Posture exercises–Exercises that improve your posture and reduce rounded or "sloping" shoulders. Posture exercises can help you decrease the risk of fractures, especially in the spine.

Quantitative computed tomography (QCT)–A test that measures bone mineral density in the spine or other bones using a CT scan and computer software. This test is less commonly used than a DXA.

Radiographic absorptiometry (RA)–A test that uses a special hand x-ray to measure bone density of the hand.

Raloxifene–The first in a class of osteoporosis medications called estrogen agonists/antagonists, which are also known as selective estrogen receptor modulators (SERMs). It is approved for women only and is taken as an oral tablet daily. The brand name is Evista®.

Registered dietitian–A resource for nutrition information and special dietary needs. Most hospitals have registered dietitians on staff and many offer outpatient instruction.

Remodeling–The ongoing process of bone formation and bone breakdown (bone loss) that occurs throughout life.

Risedronate–A medication that can prevent and treat osteoporosis in women and men. It is in a class of medications called bisphosphonates. It is taken as an oral tablet daily, weekly, twice monthly or monthly. The brand name is Actonel®.

Reclast®–See zoledronic acid.

Resistance or strengthening exercises–Exercises that help to build and maintain bone density. These exercises include lifting weights, using elastic exercise bands, weight machines or lifting your own body weight.

Resorption–The process of bone breakdown and loss.

Rheumatoid arthritis–An autoimmune disease in which the membrane surrounding the joints becomes inflamed. Steroid medications that are often used to reduce inflammation, as well as the condition on its own, can increase the risk of osteoporosis.

Risk factor–Anything that is known to make you more likely to have a certain problem. For osteoporosis, risk factors include low bone mineral density, low body weight, family history of fractures, a previous fracture and smoking.

SERM–See Estrogen agonist/antagonist.

Single energy x-ray absorptiometry (SXA)–A test used to assess bone density in the wrist or forearm.

Steroids–See corticosteroids.

Support group–A group of people who come together to share common concerns. An osteoporosis support group can allow you to express feelings and fears and share ideas for coping with the disease.

Teriparatide–The first in a class of osteoporosis medications called anabolics. It is a type of parathyroid hormone. It works by helping to form new bone. Teriparatide is taken as a daily injection by the patient. The brand name is Forteo®.

T-score–A number that shows the amount of bone you have in comparison to a healthy young adult.

Testosterone–The main male sex hormone. In men, testosterone protects bone. Low levels of the hormone can lead to bone loss.

Ultrasound densitometry–A test that uses sound waves to assess bone density in the heel.

Vertebrae–The 33 bones that form the spinal column, or backbone.

Vertebroplasty–A procedure in which bone cement is injected into recently fractured vertebrae to relieve persistent or severe pain.

Vitamin D–A vitamin formed in the skin when it is exposed to sunlight. Vitamin D helps the body use calcium to keep bones strong. It is available in a few foods such as fortified milk and cereal, egg yolks and fatty fish.

Weight-bearing, impact exercises–Exercises that help to build and maintain bone density. These exercises include activities that make you move against gravity while being upright, such as fast walking, running, stair climbing and playing soccer.

Z-score–A number that shows the amount of bone you have in comparison to other people of your age group, gender and weight.

Zoledronic acid–A medication that can treat osteoporosis in women. It is in a class of medications called bisphosphonates. It is given once a year by intravenous (IV) infusion over at least 15 minutes. The brand name is Reclast®.

Acknowledgements

Established in 1984, the National Osteoporosis Foundation (NOF) is the nation's leading voluntary health organization solely dedicated to osteoporosis and bone health.

National Osteoporosis Foundation's Vision: To make bone health a reality and a lifelong priority for all individuals.

National Osteoporosis Foundation's Mission: To prevent osteoporosis and related fractures, to promote lifelong bone health, to help improve the lives of those affected by osteoporosis and to find a cure through programs of awareness, advocacy, public and health professional education and research.

Statement of Editorial Independence

In order to accomplish our mission—to prevent osteoporosis and related fractures, to promote lifelong bone health, to help improve the lives of those affected by osteoporosis and to find a cure—NOF accepts support from diversified sources, including individual donors, memberships, sales of educational materials, investment income and grants from foundations, government sources and corporations.

While some of these funds may be restricted to specific projects, NOF maintains its independence and objectivity in accordance with the National Health Council's guiding principles. Grants accepted from corporations, which include companies involved in healthcare and consumer products and services, are accepted only on an unrestricted basis. This means that NOF alone determines the ideas and content published or promoted in the program created by grant support.

All of the educational resources produced by NOF are developed and/or reviewed by independent experts selected for their knowledge about a particular subject. Scientific members of NOF's Board of Trustees, as well as other leading experts in the field of osteoporosis, are routinely consulted to provide a fair and balanced perspective regarding written materials and educational programming.

NOF policy ensures that its recommendations are consistent with positions of the National Institutes of Health, findings of the U.S. Food and Drug Administration, guidelines of relevant medical societies, and professional consensus statements or evidence-based research published in peer reviewed journals. NOF does not endorse any particular product, service or point of view. NOF does, however, inform the public about all FDA-approved therapies, as well as the availability of other appropriate products and services, as part of its educational responsibility to the public and healthcare professionals.

NOF recommends that when using treatments for osteoporosis, as with all medications, individuals follow the instructions provided by their healthcare provider and presented in the package insert for that medication. It is important that the patient tell the doctor about any other drugs he or she is taking, including non-prescription medicines and alcohol. If a serious side effect occurs, the patient should immediately report the event to the healthcare provider and inquire about stopping the medication.

NOF is in full compliance with the Good Operating Practices and meets the Standards of Excellence of the National Health Council, meets the strong and comprehensive standards of the Better Business Bureau's Wise Giving Alliance and has been awarded the Independent Charities Seal of Excellence.

Acknowledgement of Support: The production and printing of this publication was made possible by an unrestricted grant from Novartis Pharmaceuticals.

Acknowledgements: This version of *Boning Up on Osteoporosis* is based upon prior versions printed in 1991, 2000, 2003 and 2005. The original handbook was prepared by the University of Connecticut Health Center, Farmington, Connecticut in collaboration with NOF.

The information included in this edition is current as of the publication date. For the most up-to-date information on osteoporosis prevention, diagnosis or treatment, consult with your healthcare provider or visit www.nof.org.

NOF wishes to acknowledge the following people for making this publication possible:

Felicia Cosman, MD
Professor of Clinical Medicine
Columbia University

Medical Director
Helen Hayes Hospital

Clinical Director, NOF

Deborah T. Gold, PhD
Associate Professor of
Medical Sociology
Departments of Psychiatry and
Behavioral Sciences, Sociology, and
Psychology and Neurosciences
Duke University Medical Center
Member, Board of Trustees, NOF
Chair, NOF Education Committee

Karen Kemmis, PT, DPT, MS, CDE
Physical Therapist
SUNY Upstate Medical University

Barbara Levin
Health Advocate
Member, Board of Trustees

Carleen Lindsey, PT, MScAH, GCS
Chief Physical Therapist
Physical Therapy and Massage
of Connecticut

Lawrence G. Raisz, MD
Director, Center for Osteoporosis
University of Connecticut
Health Center
Member, Board of Trustees, NOF

Mehrsheed Sinaki, MD
Mayo Clinic
Department of Physical Medicine
and Rehabilitation

Boning Up was originally
developed by the UConn Center
for Osteoporosis, part of the New
England Musculoskeletal Institute at
the University of Connecticut Health
Center in Farmington.

Current staff of the Center are:
Lawrence Raisz MD, Director
Wendy Tolman Andrews, MS
Lisanne Cirullo, APRN
Joseph Lorenzo, MD
Pooja Luthra, MD
Faryal Mirza, MD
JoAnne Smith MD,
  Clinical Director
Pamela Taxel, MD

NOF Staff Members

Judy Chandler, MPH
Project Leader
Health Education Specialist,
Education, NOF

Sandra Lockhart, RN, BSN
Manager, Health Education, NOF

Susan Randall, RN, MSN, FNP-BC
Senior Director, Education, NOF

Leo Schargorodski
Executive Director and CEO, NOF

Carol Beers
Receptionist, Finance and
Administration, NOF

Audrey Shively, MSHSE, CHES
Manager, Research and
Education, NOF

Harriet Shapiro, MA, RN
Director of Patient and Professional
Education, NOF
(retired)

Other Contributors

Mary Anne Dunkin
Freelance Writer

Kelly Trippe, MA
NOF Consultant

Reviewers

Felicia Cosman, MD
Deborah T. Gold, PhD
Karen Kemmis, PT, DPT, MS, CDE
Barbara Levin
Lawrence G. Raisz, MD